WHOLE FOOD PLANT-BASED

COOKBOOK

365 DAYS OF SUPER EASY PLANT-BASED RECIPES FOR CLEAN & HEALTHY EATING

BY SAMANTHA GREEN

TABLE OF CONTENTS

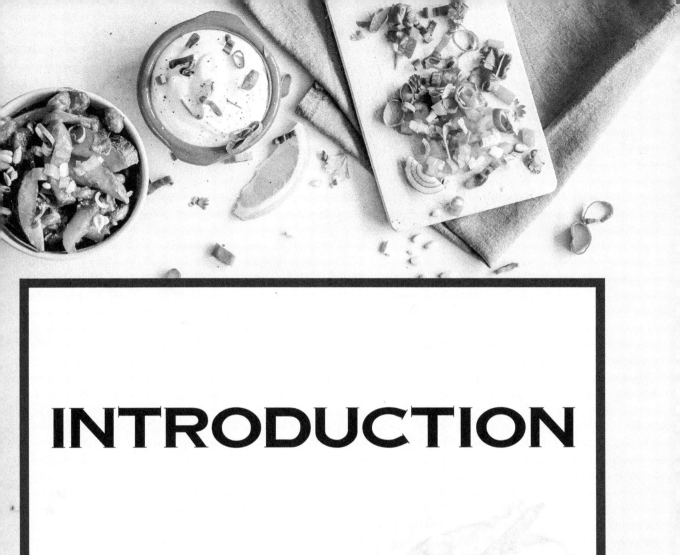

INTRODUCTION

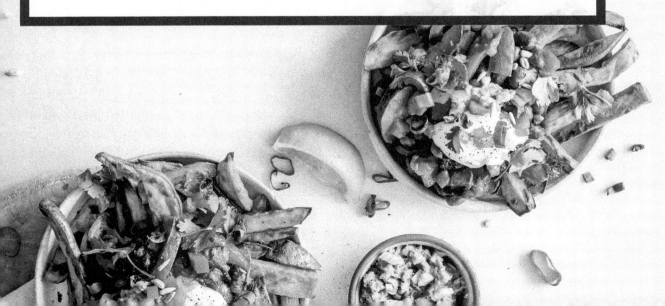

Until I went on a whole-food, plant-based (WFPB) diet three years ago, I had reasoned myself into explanatio for each decade of my increasing inability to lose weight. In my late twenties it was a sluggish metabolis broken by continuous efforts to diet myself into waif-thinness like my idol Kate Moss. I took it too far or too lor and for far too many times.

In my thirties and forties I blamed hormone imbalances for my resistant weight gain. It had to be the bi control pills, then pregnancy and later, menopause, which we know slows our metabolism even more. That mu explain the fact that no matter what diet I tried, if I lost any weight it all came right back, I thought.

What I did not know until I started this life-saving and utterly delicious way of eating, is that I had a toxic bo from years of eating diet foods, frozen foods, convenience foods (dressings, condiments, etcetera) and fast fo - the big killer, full of nasty trans fats and MSG.

And it wasn't until my doctor told me that I was at risk for diabetes that I began to take the situation seriously – serious as the look in his eyes when he told me.

THE SMARTEST DOCTOR I KNOW WEIGHS IN . . .

I had tried pretty much every diet imaginable. Some of the main diets I tried were low-fat, super low-calorie (f around 15 years), Atkins (2 years on and off, or as long as I could stand the deprivation) and most recently, t ketogenic diet. All I thought about was corn and tomato casserole, broccoli and cauliflower with Italian seasonir sliced tomatoes, tomato sauce, ratatouille, squash, eggplant, sweet potatoes the entire time. I felt sick from t lack of fresh fruit and vegetables providing me with those all important micronutrients and antioxidants.

So, at this point I asked my family physician, an 81-year-old family practitioner and internal medicine special - a man who stays more up to date on the latest science on everything related to nutrition than any doctor I' ever met - what he thought the problem could be. He had known me for over 20 years. He knew my type personality, my steely determination, how I could do anything I set my mind to . . If I was this strong perso then why couldn't I lose weight and be rid of this body shame? Why?

"Why," I said, starting to cry with humiliation, "Why must I have this huge, flabby flat tire around my belly?? W do I always feel so tired yet still get such bad sleep?? I've tried everything! Low-fat, keto, Atkins, even hormon balancing diets and hormone patches."

Dr. B replied, "It's toxins, dear. That belly there and those energy levels. That's inflammation. Your body hol water to dilute the toxic fluids within in a 50/50 fashion to keep you alive. That's called fluid retention ar inflammation. The more toxins, the more inflammation. . . That's not fat," he said tapping the tire with his pe "that's inflammation . . . You need to try eating a clean diet – greens, no hormone-injected meats, no mercu loaded fish or seafood, no sugar, no processed foods, no white refined anything . . . If you must drink coffee, g mycotoxin-free coffee that is single sourced from one grower, one crop . . . And give up anything with the wor "diet", aspartame, 'lite'. Eat whole, plant-based . . . Everything is clean. And filter your water. You'll lose that spa tire and regain your health! And for good! Just watch what happens." He added, "And read How Not to Die. promise – you won't want to eat meat after that. And the more you educate yourself, the easier it will be to sti to this diet."

HE POISONS IN OUR DIET

know now that any kind of diet without vegetables is simply ludicrous.

ne of the biggest reasons you need plants and the nutrients they contain is for detoxifying the body.

ee, our liver and kidneys can only handle so much. What the liver cannot recognize, say perfluorocarbons om a Teflon pan, it sends to the kidneys. The kidneys are these fragile little things. They cannot handle BIG oisons.

ey send these back to the liver going "No. I don't think we should send these through." The liver then alizes, hey, I've got nowhere to flush this. So might as well store it in the fat tissue till we figure this out."

e very reason we cannot detoxify these poisons that are coming into our bodies every single day is that we ck the minerals from vegetables that the liver needs to combine with these poisons to render them safe.

e liver uses things like phytonutrients to combine with toxins and then dilutes them enough to be safe for e kidneys. But if we're not eating those minerals in plants like kale, spinach, and beet greens, we have no aterials to dilute them with.

o, we must have vegetables with all of their nutritious compounds or our bodies won't be able to remove ren basic toxins. Furthermore, a diet of meat and nothing else but meat means a body full of hormones that e hard-wired to make you fat, which is exactly what they give our cattle - hormones to plump them up in the rst place!

t the bottom, the real problem was that I was ingesting a diet of poisons. And poisons do not only make you ck, they inflame your entire body. Just as if you'd gotten bitten by a snake on your ankle so your ankle puffs p to prevent the poison from reaching the heart .. But what if the poisons come in the stomach and go into e bloodstream and the cells? Well, picture ingesting that venom. Then your whole body puffs up.

ok at conventionally raised poultry, for example. Farmers actually give these chickens arsenic in their feed set off the very inflammatory response I'm speaking of. When chickens eat this feed, they puff up, like a utterball turkey. Not the skinny, feathered things they really are. If you don't believe me on this, just do a uick Google search and you will see exactly what I'm talking about.

o, imagine what that does for our weight and more importantly, our health?

UCCEEDING ON THE WFPB DIET

When I switched to the Whole Foods Plant-Based Diet (WFPB) my life changed completely. Not overnight, mind you. The goal of the diet is to detoxify the body so it can lose weight again and to give your body the vitamins and minerals it needs that are causing these cravings for sweets, breads, fast food, and processed foods so that you can finally win the fight for your health and get a slim, sleek, beautiful body!

WHAT'S DIFFERENT ABOUT THIS DIET?

I began eating plant-based, whole foods only and buying organic whenever I could, especially when purchasing any Dirty Dozen vegetables that are voted most toxic by the EWG.

And for the first time in my life, I found a diet that did the opposite of all the other diets.

Where they failed, the WFPB Diet succeeded. I lost 45 pounds, and kept it off (so far 2 years).

While other diets made me feel tired and depleted, the WFPB made me feel lighter and more energetic with each day that passed.

While other diets caused brain fog and forgetfulness, the WFPB diet helped me stay focused and get more done in less time, leaving me more hours to enjoy my life every day!

If you follow this diet, detoxify your life and your food, filter your water, avoid toxic chemicals in the home, and most of all eat the rainbow – a full spectrum of multi-colored vegetables and fruits, you will discover a life of happiness, health, and renewal that you have never experienced before.

SO, JUST WHAT IS THE WHPB DIET?

Whole foods are simply foods in their unchanged form. An ear of corn. A stalk of broccoli. A bell pepper. container of whole oats.

Therefore, a whole-food, plant-based diet focuses on plants in their original form. Opting for whole-grain oa over say, Quaker Instant Oatmeal. Grabbing the freshly squeezed orange juice in the fridge instead of the o in a box on the shelf.

In other words, nothing in a box, bottle or can that contains preservatives, colorings, flavorings or artific ingredients.

For example, buying apples and cinnamon and making your own applesauce instead of store-bought applesau filled with preservatives (or buying a jar of organic, unsweetened applesauce without any other ingredients.

Buying Extra Virgin Olive Oil (EVOO) and Bragg's Apple Cider Vinegar (with the mother) and making your ov oil and vinegar dressing instead of buying Kraft's Oil and Vinegar salad dressing.

But most of all the whole-food, plant-based diet is about avoiding hormone-injected cattle, arsenic-fed chicke and their eggs, milk filled with RBS-t and other dangerous chemicals and avoiding dangerous dyes, foo preservatives, food-colorings, flavor-enhancers, mycotoxins, excitotoxins, and chemicals in general – so th you can live a full, healthy, happy life and one free from many diseases caused by inflammation.

Ultimately, most of us are not Madonna. We can't afford salmon shipped from the cleanest portions of t Mediterranean Sea daily to keep ourselves healthy and youthful. Although this certainly has worked for h most of us are not billionaires. We must do what we can to eat clean. That's the key. Eating whole and clean.

We must do what we can to preserve our own bodies, youth, and health.

WHAT COOKING OIL SHOULD I USE?

I believe in olive oil. Extra-virgin, first-cold pressed when I can afford it, coconut oil when I cannot. For frying, when I want to make, say, rice paper rolls stuffed with vegetables or fried potatoes of any kind, I use grapeseed oil. It has a high smoking point and lots of nutrient-dense oleic acid.

What's important is to avoid industrial seed, vegetable and animal based oils at all costs

I have studied the Blue Zones – the five areas of the world where people live the longest. People that live in, say, Sardinia, Italy, for example, consume olives and olive oil daily and most live from somewhere between 105 and 115 years old.

Some may choose to cook without olive oil or add it to your salads. Here is my problem with people on the WFPB diet who say they'd rather use a non-stick skillet and fry their vegetables without oil. That non-skillet will cause more harm to your body through dangerous chemicals. Teflon, the chief chemical found in most non-stick cookware, is a known cancer-causing agent and the fumes from these pans have been shown to kill birds in numerous studies!

Just making the change to a plant-based diet alone is life-saving. So, I say, let's not be too restrictive with plant-based oils. Avocado, olive, and coconut oils have all been proven healthy and we must have fat in our diet in order to absorb fat-soluble vitamins in the first place. Without butter, I believe we need that oil for our eyes, skin, hair, cells . . . without fat, our bodies cannot thrive. But it is of utmost importance that we buy high quality plant oils.

ON SALT . . .

I believe in salt. Our bodies cannot manufacture minerals the way that they manufacture, say, vitamin D in reaction to the sun. Lysine, for example, which our body needs as one of the building blocks of protein and to transform our energy from amino acids into ATP (our cellular fuel), is only obtained from comets hitting the Earth. They say we might all be stardust. .. well, there you go!

Our soils are so over-tilled, stripped, and depleted, many of us are not getting the minerals we need even from organic vegetables and fruits. For more on this, see the Donald Davis' study titled on how minerals in vegetables have drastically dropped from 20 to 55% in all vegetables since 1950.

So mineral-replacing sources that help us make food palatable that are clean and not loaded with preservatives, I feel, are quite allowable. These include Himalayan Pink Salt and sea salt, both in moderation.

HOW IS A PLANT-BASED DIET DIFFERENT THAN THE AMERICAN FOOD PYRAMID

The food pyramid does not distinguish between a bad starch and one that comes from a box, bottle or can. It also fills your plate with starches, not necessarily healthy ones, to the detriment of vegetables. The whole-food, plant-based diet focuses solely on healthy plants, specifically fruits, vegetables, tubers, and legumes, in their purest form affordable (or available) as the sole source of nutrition for all meals.

Furthermore, the Standard American Diet (SAD) is composed almost entirely of foods that lack phytonutrien and antioxidants–the compounds we require to prevent premature aging, dementia, inflammation, and canc Sweeteners, animal products, refined grains, and manmade industrial seed oils all lack these too. In fact, the SA only get 2% of its nutrition from vegetables.

HOW IS A PLANT-BASED DIET DIFFERENT THAN A VEGAN OR VEGETARIAN DIET?

Vegan diets exclude all animal products but still allow for sweets, refined flours and other foods that contain toxin Vegetarian diets typically allow dairy products and sweets, refined flours, white bread and other manmade foo that are full of artificial ingredients that may harm health. Think of the whole-food, plant-based diet as the cleane vegan diet possible.

WHAT ARE THE BENEFITS OF A WHOLE-FOOD, PLANT-BASED DIET?

According to the most reliable and recent science, a whole-food, plant-based diet has proven to:

- Improve or even reverse cardiovascular disease
- Improve, prevent, or even reverse type II diabetes,
- Help patients to lose or maintain weight
- Prevent, improve, or reverse inflammation
- Prevent the development of neurodegenerative diseases

WHEN WILL I SEE BENEFITS/CHANGES IN MY BODY/APPEARANCE ON A WFPB DIET?

You will be able to feel a change in your body–your energy, mood, and motivation – even the same day, both I and most who follow the diet will tell you. I started to lose weight after about 2 months in on the diet. But my body was saturated with artificial sweeteners from being on diet coke and coffee with Sweet and Low or Equal since the age of 14. So . . . the more polluted the tissue, the longer it takes to get the bad guys out that are trapping water in the body to protect you from cell-poisoning.

Most people say they feel better immediately–lighter, more energetic . . . Most people lose weight at a rate of abou a pound or more a week and most claim to drop around 10 pounds the first month.

WHY THE RECIPES IN THIS BOOK ARE DIFFERENT

This book is full of recipes I learned from other chefs while I was in cooking school.

In fact, the food you'll find in this book is far too delicious to be called diet food. You shouldn't think of eating whol food, plant-based as any kind of deprivation diet but as a celebration of health and flavor. Instead of feeling ove stuffed and uncomfortably full after a meal, you'll feel satiated, but not overfull, and energized instead of tired.

ctually went to cooking school after discovering how much the whole-food, plant-based diet changed my life. I knew ot about cooking meat-based dishes, but I knew little about the cooking of vegetables, besides the usual dish of ttered corn or green beans cooked with ham. How could I make them taste better without ham, I wondered?

us, I wanted to be able to cook international dishes like Indian curries, Japanese stir fries and Chinese soups. I nted to know how to use all these fragrant curry pastes and spices to impart flavor because:

. I had started to lose weight and regain my health with the WFPB diet and wanted to stick with it

. I knew I couldn't do that without keeping it exciting, interesting, and flavorful

  I wanted to know the macronutrient ratios to use so I could create real recipes to share with others online. By doing this I knew I could save lives and help people discover a new way to live longer, lose weight, and get off medications that were polluting their bodies - making them inflamed and overweight.

, I enrolled at a cooking school and got a personal chef degree. In every class I took, I was so enthusiastic to learn at the chefs always gave me the vegetarian option to cook and coached me when I had questions or faltered. And ey started bringing me their favorite recipes.

en, I really started learning about cooking.

turns out a lot of chefs are vegetarian. They have to taste and cook so often, they've seen many chefs get horribly erweight and die far too young. They too had found that a vegetarian or vegan diet allowed them to stay thinner d energetic, even though most of them stand some 16 hours a day.

, I learned a lot about cooking whole, plant-based foods in new and exciting ways that keep this diet exciting, and e shared them all with you!

you're ready for some of the most delicious chef-created recipes you've ever eaten – so good you'll never even miss eat again – just turn the page. Get ready to feel lighter, more energetic, more glowing than you've ever felt, all while sing weight yet never feeling hungry – just turn the page!

A QUICK FOOD GUIDE

Here are some of the foods that make up the base of the WFPB diet. Eat freely, eat in moderation or avoid

EAT FREELY	IN MODERATION	AVOID
These are Whole Foods that are not processed and are as natural as possible	These are Plant-Based foods that have been minimally processed and are higher in fat	Highly processed foods, refined sugar and animal products
Fruits: *berries, citrus, melons, stone fruit, apples, banana's etc.* **Vegetables:** *potatoes, broccoli, beets, carrots, zucchini, leafy greens, etc.* **Mushrooms:** *porcini, portabello, oyster, shiitake, button etc.* **Whole Grains:** *rice, oats, barley, quinoa, buckwheat, etc.* **Legumes:** *black beans, lentils, Chickpeas, green peas, etc.* **Herbs & Spices:** *cinnamon, turmeric, cayenne pepper, chilli, basil, thyme, ginger, rosemary*	**Good Fats:** *nuts, seeds, avocado, nut butters, tahini* **Lightly Processed Food:** *whole-grain flour, tofu, whole-grain pasta* **Unsweetened plant-based milks:** *almond milk, rice milk, oat milk* **Condiments:** *vinegar, mustard, miso, fermented foods* **Natural Sweeteners:** *maple syrup, date paste, coconut sugar, honey*	**Meat:** *chicken, beef, pork, lamb, venison* **Seafood:** *fish, shellfish, shrimp* **Dairy:** *milk, cheese, yoghurt, cream, whey, ghee, butter* **Eggs** **Processed vegan foods:** *processed meat alternatives, packaged snacks, processed premade meals, vegan ice cream*

21 DAY MEAL PLAN

B. Breakfast **L.** Lunch **D.** Dinner

DAY 1	DAY 2	DAY 3	DAY 4	DAY 5	DAY 6	DAY 7
B. Quinoa Nut Berry Porridge **L.** Lettuce Bean Burritos **D.** Black Bean Burgers	**B.** Healthy Pancakes with Fruit **L.** Quinoa Kale Bowl **D.** Portabella Bourguignon	**B.** Avocado Tofu Tacos **L.** Easy Italian Bowl **D.** Vegan Gluten-Free Pizza	**B.** Pear Oatmeal Casserole **L.** Sweet Olive Salad **D.** Three Bean Chili	**B.** Sweet Potato Breakfast **L.** Mango Chutney Wraps **D.** Vegan Pot Pie	**B.** Pumpkin Pie Pancakes **L.** Cooked Cauliflower Bowl **D.** Spicy Vegetable Curry	**B.** Scrambled Tofu and Veggies **L.** Vegetable Herb Salad **D.** Sweet Potato Nachos

DAY 8	DAY 9	DAY 10	DAY 11	DAY 12	DAY 13	DAY 14
B. Healthy Tofu Tacos **L.** Mediterranean Raw Salad **D.** Cabbage Quinoa Stew	**B.** Spiced Vegan Sausage **L.** Black Bean Taquitos **D.** Sweet Potato Noodles	**B.** Multi-Grain Porridge **L.** Vegetable Tacos **D.** Cabbage Curry and Chickpeas	**B.** Tomato Tofu Bake **L.** Lettuce Bean Burritos **D.** Thick Cauliflower Rice Soup	**B.** Eggless Vegetable Quiche **L.** Fennel Cabbage Salad **D.** Black Bean Burgers	**B.** Quinoa Nut Berry Porridge **L.** Quinoa Kale Bowl **D.** Thai Curry Stew	**B.** Apple Pie Pancake **L.** Spicy Cabbage Salad **D.** Portabella Bourguignon

DAY 15	DAY 16	DAY 17	DAY 18	DAY 19	DAY 20	DAY 21
B. Avocado Tofu Tacos **L.** Mediterranean Raw Salad **D.** Vegetable Fajita Soup	**B.** Sweet Potato Tofu Hash **L.** Easy Italian Bowl **D.** Delicious Vegan Tacos	**B.** Pear Oatmeal Casserole **L.** Cooked Cauliflower Bowl **D.** Vegan Pot Pie	**B.** Scrambled Tofu and Veggies **L.** Black Bean Taquitos **D.** Spicy Vegetable Curry	**B.** Pumpkin Pie Pancakes **L.** Lettuce Bean Burritos **D.** Filling Squash Bowls	**B.** Autumn Apple Muffins **L.** Mango Chutney Wraps **D.** Vegan Enchiladas	**B.** Eggless Vegetable Quiche **L.** Quinoa Kale Bowl **D.** Coconut Curry

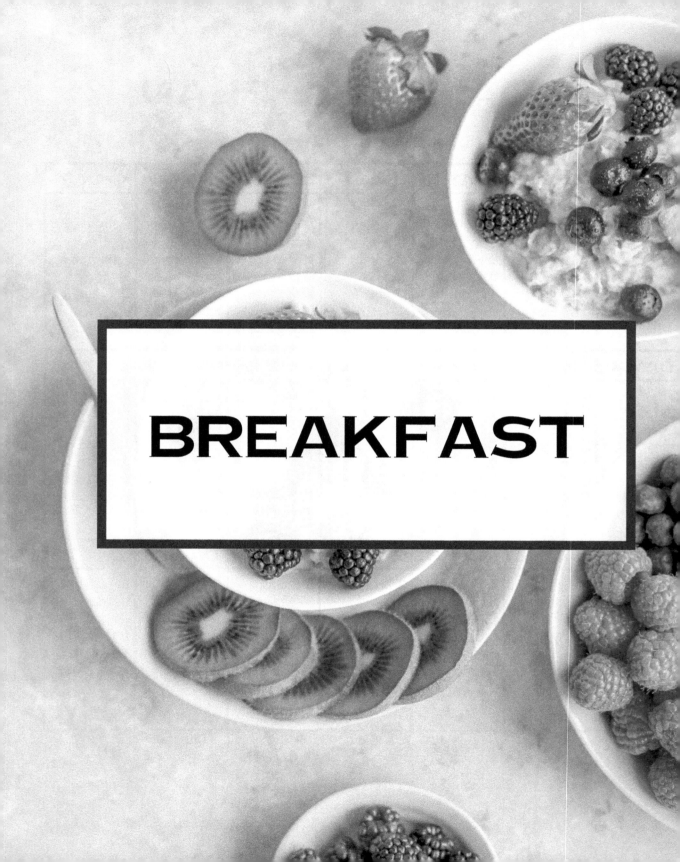

BREAKFAST

QUINOA NUT BERRY PORRIDGE

COOK TIME: 26 MINS | SERVES 6

INGREDIENTS:

- 1 cup water
- 1/8 tsp. sea salt
- 1 cup white quinoa
- 1 ½ cup oat milk
- 1 cup mixed berries
- ½ cup sliced and toasted pecans
- 1 tbsp. agave

DIRECTIONS:

1. Put the water and salt in a pot and bring to a boil.

2. Add quinoa and reduce to medium heat. Cover the pot and simmer for 16 minutes, or until quinoa is softened.

3. Stir in the milk and continue simmering, stirring every few minutes until the milk is thoroughly mixed in and quinoa is thick and soft. This will take around 10 minutes.

4. Take pot off heat and add your berries, nuts, and sweetener to taste.

Healthy Pancakes with Fruit

COOK TIME: 10 MINS | SERVES 6

INGREDIENTS:

- 1 ½ cups whole wheat flour
- ¼ cup corn flour
- ¼ cup oats or oat flour
- 1 tbsp. baking powder
- ½ tsp. salt
- ¼ tsp. ground cinnamon
- 1/8 tsp. ground nutmeg
- 1/8 tsp. ground cardamom
- 1 ¾ cups oat milk
- ½ smooth applesauce
- 2 tbsp. agave
- 1 cup strawberries (for topping)
- Honey (for topping)

DIRECTIONS:

1. Preheat the oven to 200°F to keep the pancakes warm.

2. Whisk all dry ingredients in a large bowl until thoroughly mixed.

3. In another bowl, whisk together your milk, applesauce, and agave.

4. Pour wet ingredients into dry ingredients and mix until just incorporated.

5. Heat a griddle or pan to medium high heat, then spoon on 1/3 cup of batter per pancake. Cook for 2-4 minutes, or until the top looks bubbly and the edges are solid. Flip and cook for another 2-4 minutes. Repeat. Place already cooked pancakes in a cooking dish in the preheated oven to keep warm.

6. Serve the warm pancakes with your sliced strawberries and honey!

SWEET POTATO TOFU HASH

COOK TIME: 30 MINS | SERVES 4

INGREDIENTS:

- 8oz tofu
- 2 sweet potatoes
- 1 large beet
- ¼ cup avocado oil
- ¾ tsp. sea salt
- ¾ tsp. black pepper

- 1 onion
- 4 cloves of garlic
- ½ tsp. chopped thyme
- 1/3 cup dairy-free heavy cream
- 2 green onions

DIRECTIONS:

1. Drain tofu by wrapping it in several layers of paper towels and leaving it with a weight on top for at least 20 minutes. Then remove tofu and cut into even pieces about ½ inch large.

2. Peel potatoes and beet, then chop both into roughly ½ inch chunks.

3. Chop onion and garlic into fine pieces and set aside.

4. Chop green onions and set aside.

5. In a large bowl, mix potato and beet pieces with 1 tbsp. oil, ½ tsp. sea salt, and ½ tsp. black pepper.

6. Cover bowl with a heat-resistant lid or plate and microwave for 10 minutes, stirring every couple minutes, until the potatoes and beet are soft.

7. While waiting for the potatoes to soften, heat a large pan over medium-high heat. Add 1 tbsp. olive oil and wait until heated.

8. Add to pan the tofu, soy sauce, ¼ tsp. sea salt, and ¼ tsp. black pepper. Leave for 4 minutes (or until one side is darkened) then flip pieces and brown the other side for another 4 minutes. Transfer to a clean bowl and set to the side.

9. Heat 2 tbsp. olive oil in the hot pan over medium high heat until hot. Add the onion, garlic, and thyme cook until the onion is translucent and soft, about 6 minutes.

10. Add to pan the microwaved veggies and creamer. Mix, then firmly press it all down into a thick pancake shape. Let it sit and cook for 2 minutes, then flip. Keep repeating for 8 minutes or until both sides are nicely browned.

11. Transfer the hash to a plate, then garnish with chopped green onions and serve.

PEAR OATMEAL CASSEROLE

COOK TIME: 40 MINS | SERVES 6

INGREDIENTS:

- 3 pears
- 2 cups oats
- ¾ cups crushed pecans
- ½ cup raisins
- ¼ cup honey
- 1 ½ tsp. ground cinnamon
- ½ tsp. ground ginger
- ¼ tsp. ground nutmeg
- ¼ tsp. cardamom
- ¼ tsp. salt
- 2 cups oat milk
- 1 tbsp. vanilla extract
- 2 tbsp. melted coconut oil

DIRECTIONS:

1. Preheat oven to 350°F. Use a 13x9 inch non-stick baking pan (or grease one with a little oil).

2. Cut pears into thin slices then evenly layer into the bottom of the pan.

3. Using a large mixing bowl, mix the oats, pecans, raisins, brown sugar, cinnamon, nutmeg, cardamom, and salt.

4. In a smaller bowl, whisk the milk, vanilla, and melted butter.

5. Add the wet ingredients to the dry ingredients and mix thoroughly.

6. Spread the mixture evenly over the pears.

7. Bake for 30-40 minutes, or until firm all the way through. Can be eaten hot or cold and saved in the fridge for several days.

AVOCADO TOFU TACOS

COOK TIME: 50 MINS | SERVES 4

INGREDIENTS:

- 14oz firm tofu
- ¼ tsp. sea salt
- ¼ tsp. black pepper
- 2 tbsp. chili powder
- 2 cans chopped tomatoes
- 4 tsp. lime juice
- 1 tbsp. honey
- 1 cup cilantro leaves

- 4 green onions
- 1 avocado
- 1 yellow onion
- 5 cloves garlic
- ½ cup canned green chilies
- ¼ cup avocado oil
- 8 taco shells or corn tortillas
- 1 lime sliced, for serving

DIRECTIONS:

1. Drain tofu by wrapping in paper towels and leaving a weight on top. Let drain for at least 20 minutes, then cut in half lengthwise before slicing into strips roughly ½ inch wide. Pat on sea salt, pepper, and ½ tsp chili powder.

2. Preheat oven to 500°F and line a large baking pan with parchment paper.

3. Save 1 ¼ cups of juice from the canned tomatoes and discard the rest. Whisk the juice with 1 tbsp. lime juice and honey. Set aside.

4. Chop cilantro, green onion, and avocado. Set aside.

5. Finely chop the onion, garlic, and green chilies then, in a mixing bowl, mix with 2 tbsp. oil, 2 tbsp. chili powder, and the tomatoes. Once mixed, pour onto the baking pan and cook for 20 minutes, then stir around and cook for another 20 minutes. It should be soft and slightly charred.

6. Bring 1 tbsp. oil to medium-high heat in a large pan on the oven. Carefully add the tofu to the hot oil and cook for 4 minutes on each side, or until browned and crispy. Remove and let drain on paper towels.

7. When the tomatoes are done cooking, move the mix to the pan and add tomato juice and bring to a simmer. Add a pinch of salt and pepper.

8. After 6 minutes, or when the sauce begins to thicken, add tofu and cook another 5 minutes.

9. While waiting, mix 1 tbsp. oil, 1 tsp. lime juice, cilantro, scallions, and avocado. Make sure everything gets evenly covered. If desired, add a pinch of salt and pepper. For extra spice, add a pinch of chili powder as well.

10. Build your taco with a layer of tofu-tomato mixture then the avocado mixture. Garnish with sliced lime and enjoy!

SWEET POTATO BREAKFAST

COOK TIME: 65 MINS | SERVES 4

INGREDIENTS:

- 4 sweet potatoes
- 1/4 cup pecans
- 1/4 cup shredded coconut
- 2 tbsp. honey
- 1 cup canned pineapple pieces
- 2 tsp. cinnamon
- ¼ tsp. salt

DIRECTIONS:

1. Preheat oven to 350°F.
2. Scrub any dirt off the potatoes before placing on a baking tray and cooking in the oven for an hour, or until the potatoes are soft. You can test this by inserting a skewer or fork.
3. While the potatoes are in the oven, chop the nuts into slices and toast in a pan over medium heat until they brown, but be careful not to burn them.
4. Combine the toasted nuts with the shredded coconut and 1 tbsp. honey. Mix thoroughly and set aside.
5. When potatoes are done cooking, cut along each on lengthwise, but leaving the halves attached.
6. Scoop out the potato, leaving enough attached to the skin to form a solid shell.
7. In a large bowl, add the potato flesh, pineapple pieces, 1 tbsp. honey, cinnamon, and salt. Stir until smooth trying to mix up any large chunks.
8. Put the potato mixture back into the potato skin, evenly divided and place back on the baking tray.
9. Evenly spread the coconut mixture on top of the potatoes and put tray back in oven for 25 minutes or until the coconut starts to brown.
10. Remove and serve!

APPLE PIE PANCAKE

COOK TIME: 35 MINS | SERVES 8

INGREDIENTS:

- 4 apples
- ¼ cup pecans.
- 1 tsp. cinnamon
- 1 tbsp. coconut oil
- ¼ cup honey
- 1 tbsp. plus 1 teaspoon fresh lemon juice
- 1½ cups all-purpose flour
- 2 tsp. baking powder
- ¼ tsp. and ⅛ tsp. salt
- 1 can coconut milk
- 2 tbsp. maple syrup
- 1 1/4 tbsp. lemon juice
- 1 ½ tsp. vanilla extract

DIRECTIONS:

1. Preheat the oven to 375°F.

2. Peel apples and thinly slice, removing the seeds.

3. Chop pecans and add to apples. Add ½ tsp. cinnamon and toss to mix.

4. In an oven-proof pan over medium heat, melt oil, then cook the apple mixture. After the apples are soft, add honey, 1 tsp. lemon juice, and a sprinkle of salt.

5. In a medium bowl, whisk together the flour, baking powder, ¼ tsp. salt, and ½ tsp. cinnamon.

6. In a new, clean bowl, mix together the coconut milk, 2 tbsp. maple syrup, 1 tbsp. lemon juice, and vanilla.

7. Add wet ingredients to dry ingredients and mix until there are no lumps.

8. Add the batter to the pan with the apples, making sure to cover everything, then put pan in the oven and bake for 35 minutes, or until fully cooked and browned.

PUMPKIN PIE PANCAKES

COOK TIME: 10 MINS | SERVES 4

INGREDIENTS:

- 2 cups whole wheat all-purpose flour
- 1 tbsp. baking powder
- 2 tsp. pumpkin pie spice
- ½ tsp. sea salt
- 2 cups oat milk
- 1 can pure pumpkin puree

- 2 eggs
- 2 tbsp. honey
- 1 tbsp. coconut oil

DIRECTIONS:

1. In a large bowl, mix flour, baking powder, pumpkin spice blend, and salt.

2. In a second bowl, combine milk, pureed pumpkin, eggs, honey, and coconut oil. Mix well.

3. Pour the liquid ingredients into the dry ingredients and stir until there are few lumps (a little is okay though

4. Heat a skillet or frying pan over medium heat and grease with a little oil. Use a measuring cup to pour 1/3 cup of batter per pancake.

5. Cook for 3 minutes, or until the batter bubbles on top and the edges are firm, then flip and cook another minutes. Repeat until all batter is used.

6. Serve with any toppings you like and enjoy!

SCRAMBLED TOFU AND VEGGIES

COOK TIME: 10 MINS | SERVES 4

INGREDIENTS:

- 14 oz tofu
- 1 bell pepper
- 1 shallot
- 1½ tsp. avocado oil
- ¾ tsp. sea salt
- 1/8 tsp. turmeric powder

- 1/8 tsp. black pepper
- 2 tbsp. basil leaves

DIRECTIONS:

1. Wrap tofu in paper towels and let drain with a weight on top. Leave for at least 20 minutes.

2. Using your hands, break apart the tofu into small chunks.

3. Finely chop bell pepper and shallot.

4. Finely chop basil and set aside.

5. In a large pan, add oil over medium-high heat. Add bell pepper and shallot. Cook for about 5 minutes or until soft.

6. Add tofu, salt, turmeric, and black pepper. Stir for another 5 or so minutes.

7. Serve and top with chopped basil.

HEALTHY TOFU TACOS

COOK TIME: 50 MINS | SERVES 4

INGREDIENTS:

- 1 lb tofu
- 1 onion
- 1 bell pepper
- 1 sweet potato
- 4 garlic cloves
- 2 tbsp. basil
- 1 tsp. thyme

- 2 tbsp. turmeric powder
- 1/4 cup nutritional yeast
- Salt
- Black pepper
- 4 wheat tortillas
- Salsa (for serving)

DIRECTIONS:

1. Wrap tofu in paper towels and let drain with a weight on top. Leave for at least 20 minutes.

2. Using your hands, break apart the tofu into small chunks.

3. Preheat oven to 350°F.

4. Finely chop onion, bell pepper, and potato.

5. In a large pan over medium heat, cook onion, bell pepper, and potato for 10 minutes, or until the potato becomes soft. Add water if needed to prevent sticking.

6. Finely chop garlic, basil, and thyme.

7. Into the pan, add garlic, basil, thyme, and turmeric. Cook another few minutes until the garlic is soft.

8. Add the crumbled tofu, nutritional yeast, salt, and pepper to the pan.

9. Transfer the pan's contents to a baking tray and spread it evenly. Cook in the oven for 35 minutes, stirring occasionally.

10. Build your burrito by filling the tortilla with the tofu mixture and topping with salsa if desired. Fold one end of the tortilla in then roll.

11. Serve with more salsa as a dip!

SPICED VEGAN SAUSAGE

COOK TIME: 30 MINS | SERVES: 10

INGREDIENTS:

- 1 tsp. sage
- ½ tsp. rosemary
- 8 oz tempeh
- 2 tbsp. honey
- 2 tbsp. whole wheat flour
- 1 tbsp. avocado oil

- 1 tbsp. red miso
- ¼ tsp. pepper
- 1/8 tsp. red pepper flakes

DIRECTIONS:

1. Preheat oven to 400°F.

2. Chop sage and rosemary.

3. Crumble tempeh into a food processor and combine with the honey, flour, oil, miso, sage, rosemary, pepper, and red pepper. Pulse until there are no large chunks.

4. Wet your hands to avoid sticking and mold the mixture into evenly sized patties.

5. Grease a large baking pan with parchment paper or non-stick oil and place the patties side by side.

6. Put pan in the oven for 15 minutes, then flip the patties and cook another 15 minutes.

7. Serve however you want!

MULTI-GRAIN PORRIDGE

COOK TIME: 10 MINS | SERVES: 4

INGREDIENTS:

- 4 cups water
- ½ cup millet
- ½ cup white quinoa
- ¼ cup amaranth
- ½ tsp. sea salt
- 1 cup oat milk

- ½ tsp. cinnamon powder
- 1/8 tsp. nutmeg powder
- 1½ cups mixed berries
- 2 tbsp. honey

DIRECTIONS:

1. Rinse the millet, quinoa, and amaranth in cold water.

2. Boil water in a large pot. Take pot off heat and mix in millet, quinoa, amaranth, and salt. Cover pot and leave to soak for 8 hours or overnight.

3. When ready to cook, mix in milk, cinnamon, and nutmeg. Place over medium heat and simmer for 10 minutes, stirring every other minute.

4. Stir in fruit and honey then serve. Keep in mind the porridge will thicken as it sits, so feel free to add more milk as needed.

EGGLESS VEGETABLE QUICHE

COOK TIME: 45 MINS | SERVES: 12

INGREDIENTS:

- 2 cups chickpea flour
- ¼ cup nutritional yeast
- 1 tsp. gluten-free baking powder
- ½ tsp. salt
- ¼ tsp. turmeric powder
- 1/8 tsp. pepper
- 2 cups spinach
- 3 cloves garlic
- 2 cups water
- 1 tbsp. avocado oil

DIRECTIONS:

1. Preheat the oven to 400°F. Grease two pie tins with oil.

2. Whisk together the flour, yeast, baking powder, salt, turmeric, and pepper in a large mixing bowl.

3. Finely chop the spinach and garlic.

4. Add the greens and garlic to the dry ingredients, then combine the water and olive oil to make a runny batter.

5. Divide the batter between the two pie tins and bake for 45 minutes, or until solid and a toothpick inserted in the middle comes out clean.

6. Let cool, slice, and serve!

TOMATO TOFU BAKE

COOK TIME: 30 MINS | SERVES: 4

INGREDIENTS:

- Two packages of tofu
- 1 onion
- 1 bell pepper
- 3 cloves garlic
- 1 tbsp. avocado oil
- 1 tbsp. red pepper paste

- ¼ tsp. turmeric powder
- 2 tbsp. tomato paste
- 1 can diced tomatoes
- 1 cup water
- ¼ tsp sea salt

DIRECTIONS:

1. Wrap the tofu in paper towels and place a weight on top. Leave to drain for at least 20 minutes before slicing into even pieces.
2. Preheat the oven to 400°F.
3. Finely chop the onion, bell pepper, and garlic.
4. Heat oil in a large frying pan over medium heat. Add the onion and cook for 5 minutes, or until onions turn transparent.
5. Add bell pepper and garlic. Cook for another 3 minutes.
6. Add red pepper paste and turmeric and cook until incorporated.
7. Add tomato paste stir for a minute or until it starts to darken.
8. Add tomatoes with juice, water, salt, and tofu into the pan and turn heat to medium-high.
9. Once the tomatoes start to bubble, transfer the contents of the pan to an oven-proof baking pan and cover with foil.
10. Cook for 15 minutes, then remove foil and cook for another 15 minutes.
11. Enjoy!

AUTUMN APPLE MUFFINS

COOK TIME: 25 MINS | SERVES: 12

INGREDIENTS:

- 1 cup whole-wheat flour
- 1 cup oat flour
- 2 tbsp. flaxseed powder
- ½ tsp. cinnamon powder
- 2 tsp. baking powder
- ½ tsp. baking soda
- ½ tsp. salt
- ½ cup honey
- ¼ cup coconut oil
- 2 eggs
- 1 tsp. vanilla extract
- 1 whole apple
- ½ cup walnuts

DIRECTIONS:

1. Preheat the oven to 350°F and line a muffin tin with paper liners or grease the cups with oil.

2. In mixing bowl, whisk together the dry ingredients.

3. In a new bowl, whisk together the honey, oil, eggs, and vanilla.

4. Pour the wet ingredients into the dry ingredients and mix until combined.

5. Peel the apple and slice into small cubes. Chop walnuts into small pieces.

6. Fold the apple and walnuts into the batter.

7. Spoon the batter evenly into the muffin tin and bake for 20 to 25 minutes, or until you can insert a skewer into the middle and it comes out clean.

8. Turn out and let cool on a wire rack before serving.

SUMMER FRUIT SMOOTHIE

COOK TIME: 4 MINS | SERVES: 2

INGREDIENTS:

- 1 orange
- 2 cups spinach
- ½ cup water
- 2 cups frozen peach pieces
- 1 frozen banana
- ½ cup sliced strawberries

- 1 peach
- 1 kiwi
- ¼ cup cashews
- 4 mint leaves

DIRECTIONS:

1. Peel the orange and slice into fourths, then add to a blender with spinach and water. Blend on high until smooth.

2. Add the frozen peaches and banana, then blend on high. If the mixture is too thick, add a little more water until you get the desired consistency and is smooth.

3. Chop the fresh fruit into slices or cubes. Chop cashews and mint leaves.

4. Spoon out the smoothie into two bowls and top with equally divided chopped fruit and cashews. Sprinkle the mint on top and serve promptly.

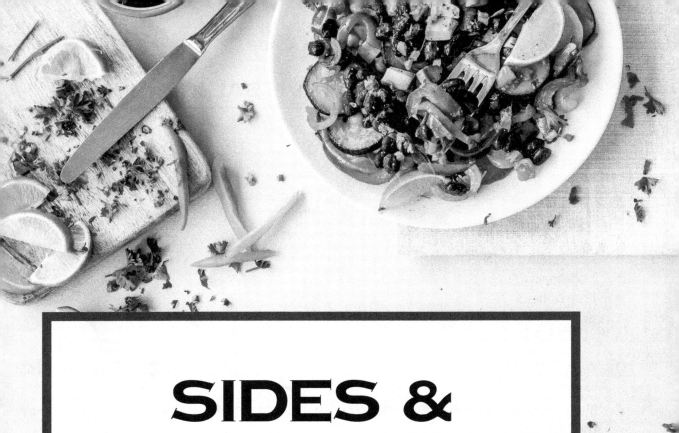

SIDES & SALADS

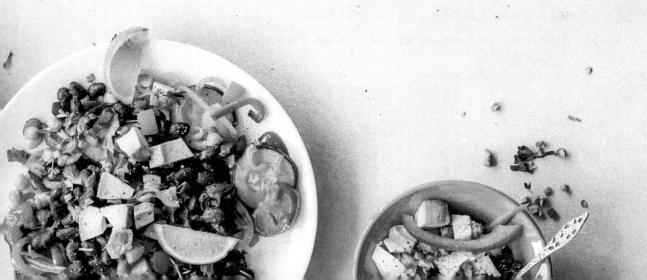

SWEET OLIVE SALAD

COOK TIME: 8 MINS | SERVES: 4

INGREDIENTS:

- 4 carrots
- 1 cup raisins
- 5 oranges
- 1 tsp. cumin powder
- 2 tsp. honey
- 1 cup cashews

- 1 cup green or black olives
- salt
- pepper

DIRECTIONS:

1. Wash and scrub the carrots to remove any dirt. Using a grater, peel the carrots into thin slivers and put aside.

2. Bring a pot of water to a boil, then place raisins into the pot. Let them soak while you prepare the rest. This adds plumpness and juice to the raisins.

3. Skin four oranges and cut them into bite-sized pieces.

4. Using a new pot, combine the orange chunks, cumin, and honey.

5. Heat the orange mixture over medium heat for 5 minutes, or until softened. Pour entire hot orange mixture over the carrots.

6. Using the empty orange pan, heat cashews over medium heat for 3-5 minutes or until browned.

7. Add cashews and olives to the carrot bowl. Drain the raisins and add those as well.

8. Squeeze the juice of the fifth orange onto the salad.

9. Sprinkle a pinch of salt and pepper over the salad, mix gently with tongs, and serve.

FENNEL CABBAGE SALAD

COOK TIME: 8 MINS | SERVES: 2

INGREDIENTS:

- 2 grapefruits
- 2 fennel bulbs
- 2 cups red cabbage
- 1 bell pepper
- 1 tbsp. fresh lime juice
- Salt

- Pepper
- ½ cup cilantro
- 1 avocado
- ¼ cup walnut

DIRECTIONS:

. Peel your grapefruits, then pith. Carefully slice the grapefruit segments out, then squeeze lightly over a large bowl. Put both fruit and juice in the large bowl.

. Thinly slice and core your fennel. Add to bowl.

. Cut the red cabbage into thin slices and add to bowl.

. Thinly slice the bell pepper and add to bowl.

. Add lime juice and a pinch of salt and pepper.

. Toss to combine.

. Just before serving, chop and add the cilantro. Top with slice avocado and chop walnuts to sprinkle on top, then serve.

QUINOA KALE BOWL

COOK TIME: 40 MINS | SERVES: 4

INGREDIENTS:

- 1 cup quinoa
- 2 cups vegetable stock
- ¼ cup raisins
- 2 tbsp. balsamic vinegar
- 1 tbsp. avocado oil
- 1 tbsp. lemon juice
- Salt

- Pepper
- 1 carrot
- 1 cup kale
- 2 scallions
- 2 tbsp. sunflower seeds
- 2 tbsp. pumpkin seeds

DIRECTIONS:

1. Rinse the quinoa in cold water, then drain.

2. In a medium pot, bring the vegetable stock to a boil.

3. Add quinoa and lower heat. Cover the pot and simmer for 20 minutes, or until the quinoa is soft all the way through.

4. To cool quinoa faster, put it in the freezer while preparing the rest of the ingredients.

5. Put the raisins in a bowl of water and let soak for at least 10 minutes.

6. Whisk together the vinegar, oil, lemon juice, a pinch of salt, and a pinch of pepper.

7. Finely chop or grate the carrot. Thinly slice kale, making sure to remove the stem, and scallions.

8. After the quinoa has cooled, move it to a large salad bowl. Add the raisins, carrot, kale, scallions, sunflower seeds, and pumpkin seeds. Top with the previously mixed dressing and toss gently to combine.

VEGETABLE HERB SALAD

COOK TIME: 45 MINS | SERVES: 4

INGREDIENTS:

- 1 butternut squash
- avocado oil
- Salt
- Pepper
- 1 tbsp. paprika powder
- 1 tbsp. Italian herb mix
- 2 bags arugula

- 1 cup black olives
- 2 avocados
- 1 tbsp. tamari
- 2 tbsp. apple cider vinegar

DIRECTIONS:

- Preheat the oven to 390°F.
- Peel the butternut squash, then cut it into pieces about an inch big.
- Spread out the squash pieces on a pan, drizzle them with oil, and generously sprinkle salt and pepper. Evenly sprinkle in paprika and dried herbs, then toss to coat.
- Cook squash for 40 minutes or until soft all the way through.
- In a small bowl, mix together the tamari, vinegar, 2 tbsp. oil, and a pinch of salt and pepper.
- Mix the arugula with the dressing and add the olives.
- Dice the avocado and add to the salad with the cooled squash. Serve.

Quick tip: This also makes an excellent warm salad if you substitute the arugula with steamed spinach!

MEDITERRANEAN RAW SALAD

COOK TIME: 5 MINS | SERVES: 2

INGREDIENTS:

- 2 romaine hearts
- 1 bell pepper
- 1 cup tomato
- ½ cup chopped cucumber
- ¼ cup chopped red onion
- 1 can of chickpeas
- ½ cup pitted Kalamata olives
- ½ container of tofu feta
- 1/3 cup cashew Tzatziki
- Pita chips
- Lemon wedges

DIRECTIONS:

1. Wash, dry, and chop the romaine hearts. Chop the bell pepper, tomato, cucumber, and red onion.
2. Add all chopped ingredients to a large bowl. Add the chickpeas and olives. Crumble feta on top.
3. Lightly drizzle with cashew tzatziki, then serve with pita chips and lemon wedges.

SPICY CABBAGE SALAD

COOK TIME: 5 MINS | SERVES: 4

INGREDIENTS:

- 1 head napa cabbage
- 1 cup carrots
- ½ cup green onions
- 1 bell pepper
- ½ cup cilantro
- 1 jalapeño chile pepper
- ½ cup sunflower seeds
- ½ cup almond butter
- ¼ cup canned coconut milk
- ¼ cup apple cider vinegar
- ¼ cup onion
- 2 tbsp. white miso paste
- 2 tbsp. honey
- 1 tbsp. red curry paste
- 3 garlic cloves
- ½-inch piece ginger

DIRECTIONS:

1. Trim the end of the cabbage, halve and core it, then cut thinly. Shred carrots, thinly slice green onions and pepper, chop cilantro and jalapeño. Combine all in a large bowl with sunflower seeds. Set aside.
2. Roughly chop onion.
3. Make the sauce by blending the almond butter, coconut milk, vinegar, onion, miso, honey, curry paste, garlic, and ginger. Blend until smooth and mixed. If needed, add water to thin it out.
4. Pour the dressing over the veggie mix and toss to coat.

WHOLESOME FARM SALAD

COOK TIME: 4 HRS | SERVES: 5

INGREDIENTS:

- 1/2 cup hulled barley
- 2 beetroots
- 2 tbsp. sunflower seeds
- 6 cups romaine lettuce
- 1/2 cup scallions
- 1/2 cup coriander
- 2 tbsp. raisins

- 1/2 cup orange juice
- 1 tbsp. lemon juice
- Black pepper
- Himalayan pink salt

DIRECTIONS:

1. In a large bowl, cover barley with water, then leave to soak for at least 3 hours.

2. Drain the barley water and add barley to a pot over high heat. Add 2 cups water and boil for 5 to 7 minutes, then turn heat to low and cover pot. Simmer 25 minutes or until the barley is tender but not soft. Drain and set aside to cool to room temperature.

3. Scrub the outside of the beets then cut each into quarters.

4. Put beets in a medium pan and add water until it covers the beets. Bring to a boil, then simmer partially covered. Simmer for 30 minutes or until the beets are tender. Drain. Peel the beets while they are still warm and cut them into bite-size pieces. Set aside.

5. Toast the sunflower seeds over medium high heat, stirring every so often, for 5 minutes or until barely toasted. Let cool on a plate.

6. Chop romaine, green onion, and cilantro.

7. In a large bowl, add the barley and beets. Add romaine, green onions, cilantro, raisins, orange juice, lemon juice, a sprinkle of pepper, and a pinch of salt. Toss gently then sprinkle the toasted sunflower seeds over the salad.

SPICY CHICKPEA CRUNCH

COOK TIME: 5 MINS | SERVES: 2

INGREDIENTS:

- 1 garlic clove
- 1 tbsp. sesame oil
- 2 tbsp. rice vinegar
- ½ tsp. hot sauce
- 2 tbsp. tamari
- 1 tsp. honey
- 2 tsp. sesame seeds
- 2 cups spinach

- 1 can chickpeas
- 2 stalks celery
- 2 carrots
- ½ cucumber
- 2 green onions
- 1 ripe avocado
- 4 tbsp. walnuts

DIRECTIONS:

1. Mince garlic and whisk with the oil, vinegar, hot sauce, tamari, honey, and sesame seeds until combined. Refrigerate until ready to serve.

2. Evenly divide the spinach between two serving bowls.

3. Drain and rinse the chickpeas, then half it between the bowls.

4. Thinly slice the celery, carrots, cucumber, green onions, and chop the avocado. Divide evenly between each bowl.

5. Thinly slice or chop walnuts and sprinkle half over each bowl. Use a measuring spoon to pour 1 tbsp. of the previously prepared dressing into each bowl and serve promptly.

CHICKPEA OLIVE MIX

COOK TIME: 25 MINS | SERVES: 6

INGREDIENTS:

- 1 cucumber, halved lengthwise, seeded, and cut into ½-inch pieces
- 1 cup grape tomatoes, quartered
- 1 tsp. salt
- 3 tbsp. red wine vinegar
- 1 garlic clove, minced
- 3 tbsp. avocado oil
- 1 can chickpeas, rinsed
- ½ cup pitted kalamata olives, chopped
- ½ red onion, chopped fine
- ½ cup chopped fresh parsley
- 2 bag spinach
- ½ cup tofu feta cheese
- ½ cup cashews

DIRECTIONS:

1. Cut cucumber into small cubes and dice tomatoes.

2. Toss cucumber and tomatoes with salt and let drain in colander for 15 minutes.

3. Mince or finely chop garlic. Chop olives, onion, and parsley.

4. In a large bowl, mix vinegar and garlic. Add and mix in the oil. Add drained cucumber-tomato mixture, chickpeas, olives, onion, and parsley. Let sit for at least 5 mins.

5. Add spinach, feta and cashews. Gently mix to coat. Season with salt and pepper to taste. Serve.

EASY ITALIAN BOWL

COOK TIME: 15 MINS | SERVES: 5

INGREDIENTS:

- 1 red onion
- 1 cup basil
- 12 ounces wheat spiral pasta
- 1 bag assorted frozen vegetables
- 1 cup balsamic vinaigrette
- Salt
- Pepper

DIRECTIONS:

1. Finely dice onion and basil.

2. Boil water in a large pot and cook pasta according to box. During the last 5 minutes of cooking, add frozen vegetables to the pot. Drain the pasta and vegetables. Rinse under cold water until cool.

3. Move mixture to a large bowl. Add the onion, vinaigrette, and basil. Gently mix to coat. Add a pinch of salt and pepper. Can be served cold or room-temperature.

LIGHT LEMON SALAD

COOK TIME: 20 MINS | SERVES: 4

INGREDIENTS:

- 1 bunch kale
- 1 bunch parsley
- 4 garlic cloves
- 2 tsp. avocado oil
- ¼ cup pitted Kalamata olives
- Grated zest and juice of 1 lemon
- Salt
- Pepper

DIRECTIONS:

1. Destem the kale, and chop finely. Roughly chop parsley and garlic.

2. Fill a pot with water and heat to medium heat. Place a steamer tray over the pot and fill it with kale, parsley, and garlic. Cover and leave for 15 minutes.

3. Add the oil to a pan over medium heat. Once the oil is hot, add the steamed greens. Cook and stir for 5 minutes.

4. Chop olives, then transfer with the greens to a bowl and add lemon zest and juice. Serve on toast with hummus and season with salt and pepper for the best experience!

Quick tip: This salad can be enjoyed cold, hot, or room temperature!

COOKED CAULIFLOWER BOWL

COOK TIME: 20 MINS | SERVES: 4

INGREDIENTS:

- 1 head cauliflower
- ½ cup avocado oil
- 1¼ tsp. salt
- 1 tsp. pepper
- 1 green onion
- 1/3 cup raisins
- 1 tsp. lemon zest
- 1 tbsp. lemon juice
- 1 tsp. coriander powder
- 1 cup parsley
- ½ cup mint
- ¼ cup sliced almonds

DIRECTIONS:

1. Adjust oven rack to lowest position and pre-heat to 475°F. degrees.
2. Cut the cauliflower into small florets. Chop and save the core of the cauliflower.
3. Add cauliflower florets, 1 tablespoon oil, 1 teaspoon salt, and ½ teaspoon pepper to a bowl. Toss to coat.
4. Transfer to baking pan and roast for 15 minutes or until florets are soft and browned on bottoms. Set aside and let cool.
5. While florets are roasting, finely chop green onion and combine with raisins, lemon zest and juice, coriander, remaining ¼ cup oil, remaining ¼ teaspoon salt, and remaining ½ teaspoon pepper in large bowl. Mix thoroughly and set aside.
6. Add cauliflower core to blender and until finely chopped. Add to the bowl with dressing.
7. Add parsley and mint to the blender and pulse until coarsely chopped. Add to bowl with dressing.
8. Finely slice almonds.
9. Add cooked cauliflower and almonds to bowl with dressing mixture and gently mix. Season with salt and pepper to taste. Serve.

SEASONED TOFU POTATO SALAD

COOK TIME: 1 HR 10 MINS | SERVES: 8

INGREDIENTS:

- 8 potatoes
- 1 package firm tofu
- 2 tbsp. yellow mustard
- 1 tbsp. Dijon mustard
- 4 cloves garlic
- 1 tbsp. fresh lime juice
- 1/2 tsp. salt

- 1/4 cup pickle relish
- 4 large stalks celery
- 1 onion
- Pepper

DIRECTIONS:

1. Roughly chop potatoes into chunks, then put in a large pot and add cold water to cover.
2. Bring to a boil then reduce heat to simmer the potatoes until just tender, 8 to 10 minutes. Drain potatoes and let cool.
3. Put the tofu, yellow mustard, Dijon mustard, chopped garlic, lime juice, and salt into a food processor and pulse until smooth and creamy.
4. Add the relish to the tofu mix and mix well.
5. Dice the celery, onion and add to the tofu bowl.
6. Chop potatoes into bite-sized pieces. Season with salt and pepper to taste. Gently mix until coated.
7. Cover bowl and refrigerate for at least 1 hour.

CLASSIC POTATO COMFORT

COOK TIME: 60 MINS | SERVES: 4

INGREDIENTS:

- 1 ½ cups long-grain rice
- 1/4 cup roasted cashews
- 4 large potatoes
- 4 cups white mushrooms
- 1 clove garlic
- 4 cups vegetable broth
- 1/2 tsp. dried sage
- 1/2 tsp. dried marjoram

- 1/2 tsp. dried thyme
- 2 tbsp. fresh lemon juice
- ½ tsp. pepper
- Salt

DIRECTIONS:

1. Cook the rice according to the package and set aside.

2. Place the cashews in a small bowl and cover with 1 cup water. Set aside to soak for 30 minutes.

3. Scrub the outside of the potatoes then chop into inch pieces. Slice the mushrooms, and finely chop garlic.

4. Place the potatoes in a pot and cover with water. Bring to a boil, then reduce heat and simmer until the potatoes are very tender when skewered, about 20 minutes. Drain and set aside to cool.

5. In a pot, combine the rice, mushrooms, and vegetable broth. Bring to a boil then reduce the heat and simmer until the mushrooms are soft, about 10 minutes. Set aside to cool.

6. Using a blender or handheld mixer, blend the mixture until smooth.

7. Put the blended mix back into the pot and add the sage, marjoram, thyme, garlic, lime juice, 1/8 teaspoon of the pepper, and a pinch of salt. Heat over medium heat for 10 minutes and stir occasionally.

8. Pour the cashews and their water into a clean blender. Add a pinch of salt and 1/4 teaspoon pepper. Blend until there are no chunks. Dump the pecan butter in a bowl with the potatoes and mash together until smooth.

9. Serve on a plate with the potatoes and gravy spooned over top.

FRIED ZUCCHINI

COOK TIME: 20 MINS | SERVES: 4

INGREDIENTS:

- 4 zucchinis
- ½ cup unsweetened almond milk
- 1 tsp. arrowroot powder
- 1 tsp. lemon juice
- ½ tsp. salt
- ½ cup panko
- ¼ cup hemp seeds
- ¼ cup nutritional yeast
- ½ tsp. garlic powder
- ¼ tsp. pepper
- ¼ tsp. red pepper flakes

DIRECTIONS:

1. Slice the zucchini into rounds.

2. Preheat the oven to 375°F and grease two large baking pans.

3. Put the zucchini in a bowl with the milk, arrowroot powder, lemon juice, and ¼ teaspoon salt. Toss to coat.

4. Mix the panko, hemp seeds, nutritional yeast, garlic powder, pepper, and crushed red pepper in a bowl. Add the zucchini in handfuls and toss to thoroughly coat.

5. Spread the zucchini in an even layer on the baking pans. Bake 20 minutes or until the zucchini is toasty.

THICK SWEET POTATO FRIES

COOK TIME: 30 MINS | SERVES: 2

INGREDIENTS:

- 2 sweet potatoes
- 1 tsp. garlic powder
- 1/2 tsp. cumin powder
- 1/2 tsp. chili powder
- 1/2 tsp. salt
- 1/2 tsp. black pepper

DIRECTIONS:

1. Preheat the oven to 425°F. Then peel and quarter sweet potatoes.

2. Fill a pot halfway with water and place over medium heat. Put a steamer tray on top and fill with the potato. Cover and steam for 8 minutes or until potatoes are softened.

3. Spread the potato evenly on a greased baking pan.

4. In a small bowl, whisk the garlic, cumin, chili powder, salt, and pepper. Sprinkle the spice mixture evenly over the sweet potatoes and toss to coat.

5. Cook for 10 minutes, then flip potatoes and cook for another 10 minutes. Potatoes should be soft and browned.

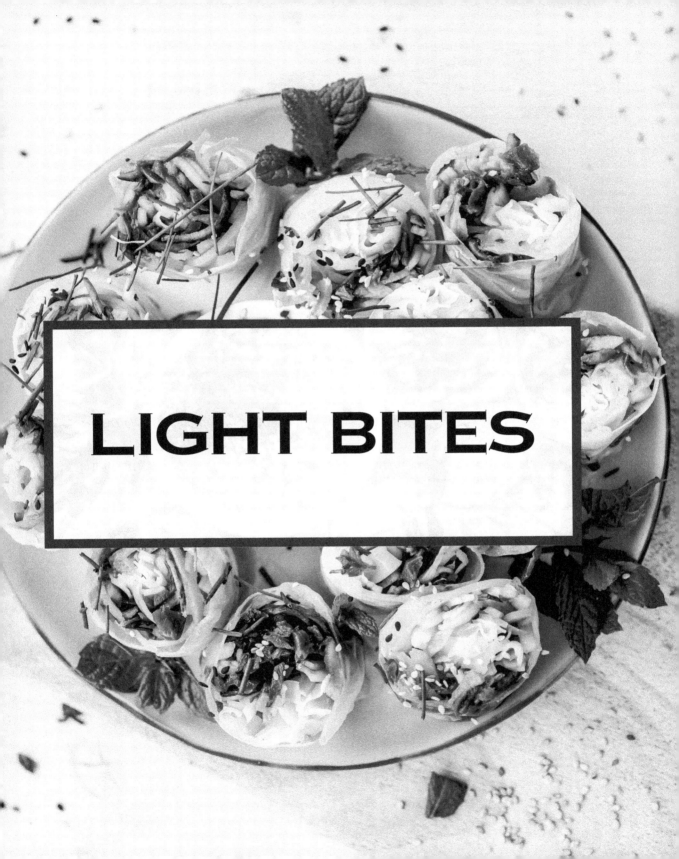

LIGHT BITES

HOT WINGS WITH RANCH

COOK TIME: 2 HRS 45 MINS | SERVES: 4

INGREDIENTS:

- ½ cup chickpea flour
- ½ cup water
- 1 tsp. garlic powder
- ½ tsp. salt
- 1 head cauliflower, chopped
- 1 tsp. avocado oil
- ²/3 cup hot sauce

- ½ cup roasted cashews
- 4 tsp. lime juice
- ½ tsp. dill
- ¼ tsp. garlic powder
- ¼ tsp. paprika
- Salt
- Pepper

DIRECTIONS:

1. Place the cashews in a bowl and add 2 tsp. of lime juice. Add enough water to cover cashews and a little more. Let soak 2 hours, then drain and rinse well.

2. In a strong blender, add cashews, ¼ cup water, dill, garlic powder, paprika, 2 tsp. lime juice, a pinch of salt, and a pinch of pepper to taste. Blend until smooth. Set aside in fridge until ready to use.

3. Preheat the oven to 450°F. Grease a large baking tray.

4. Chop the cauliflower into bite-sized florets.

5. Whisk together the flour, water, garlic powder, and salt.

6. Dip the florets in the batter, coating each piece thoroughly. Place carefully on the baking tray and cook for 8 minutes. Flip florets over and cook another 8 minutes.

7. While the cauliflower is cooking, whisk together the oil and hot sauce.

8. When the cauliflower is done, move the florets to the bowl with the sauce and coat thoroughly. Place the sauce-covered cauliflower back on the baking sheet and cook for 25 minutes or until crispy.

9. Serve the cauliflower with cold sauce.

BREADED TEMPEH BITES

COOK TIME: 35 MINS | SERVES: 4

INGREDIENTS:

- 8 oz package tempeh
- ¼ cup oat milk
- ¼ cup nutritional yeast
- 1 tbsp. pre-blended spice mix
- 1 tsp. arrowroot powder
- 1 tsp. fresh lime juice

- ¼ tsp. pepper
- ¼ tsp. hot sauce
- ¼ tsp. salt
- 1 cup panko

DIRECTIONS:

Preheat the oven to 400°F. Grease a large baking pan.

Cut the tempeh in half and cut into 8 pieces. Squish each piece lightly to flatten slightly.

In a bowl, combine the milk, nutritional yeast, seasoning blend, arrowroot powder, lime juice, pepper, hot sauce, and salt. Add the tempeh bits and let soak for 5 minutes. Make sure each piece is evenly coated.

Pour the panko on a plate. Dip each piece of tempeh from the batter to roll in the panko. Place on the prepared baking pan.

Cook for 15 minutes. Flip all pieces, then cook for another 15 minutes or until golden brown.

CUMIN CHILI CHICKPEAS

COOK TIME: 45 MINS | SERVES: 6

INGREDIENTS:

- 1 can chickpeas
- 1 tbsp. paprika powder
- 1 tbsp. cumin powder
- 2 tsp. red chili flakes
- 2 tbsp. honey
- 3 tbsp. lemon juice
- 1 tbsp. avocado oil
- Sea salt
- Black pepper

DIRECTIONS:

1. Preheat oven to 395°F.
2. Drain and rinse the chickpeas, then spread them on a large oven pan.
3. Mix together the paprika, cumin, chili flakes, and a pinch of salt and pepper. Evenly powder over the chickpeas.
4. Mix together the honey, lemon juice, and oil, then pour over the chickpeas. Stir the mixture to make sure the chickpeas are fully coated.
5. Cook for 45 minutes, or until browned and crisp.

Quick tip: Use these delicious chickpeas on your salads!

SUMMER SUSHI

COOK TIME: 10 MINS | SERVES: 6

INGREDIENTS:

- 2 cucumbers
- 2 avocados
- 4 tbsp. lime juice
- 2 tbsp. extra-virgin olive oil
- Sea salt
- Black pepper

DIRECTIONS:

- Peel the cucumber skin off and throw it away.
- Peel or slice each cucumber length-wise, going from the bottom to the top. Discard the very middle of the cucumber, as it is not strong enough to shape.
- After the cucumbers are sliced, take each slice and tightly roll it from the bottom up.
- Cut open the avocado and discard the pit. Cut the avocado flesh into tiny squares and put inside the cucumber circles. Cram as much in as possible for a more stable roll.
- After you've completed your rolls, lightly cover with lime juice and olive oil. Sprinkle a pinch of salt and pepper on top and serve!

SPECIAL CHEESE BOARD

COOK TIME: 30 MINS | SERVES: 8

INGREDIENTS:

- 2 cups almond flour
- 4 tbsp. onion powder
- Water
- 1 tsp. light soy sauce
- 1 tbsp. poppy seeds
- 5 tsp. agar agar powder
- ½ cup bell pepper
- ½ cup raw cashews

- 1 ⅓ cup nutritional yeast
- 4 tbsp. lemon juice
- ½ tsp. mustard

DIRECTIONS:

1. Preheat the oven to 350°F.

2. To make the crackers, mix together the flour, 3 tbsp. onion powder, 3 tbsp. water, soy sauce, and poppy seeds. Form into a ball.

3. Cover a baking tray with parchment paper and place the ball on top. Press it down as flat as possible, the place another piece of parchment sheet on top.

4. On top of the second sheet of parchment, use a rolling pin to roll the cracker mix to about 1/4th inch thick.

5. Remove the second sheet of parchment and cook in oven for about 15 minutes.

6. When the crackers are done baking, let cool and cut into cracker-sized pieces. Store in an airtight container.

7. Put the agar agar and 1 ½ cups of water into a small pot over high heat. Wait for it to boil and whisk continuously until the mixture becomes thick like custard.

8. Remove from heat and scoop into a blender.

9. Roughly chop pepper and add to the blender along with the cashews, nutritional yeast, lemon juice, 2 tsp. onion powder, and mustard. Pulse until smooth.

10. Pour the blended mix into a bread pan lined with parchment paper and refrigerate for at least 30 minutes before serving.

3-INGREDIENT FLATBREAD

COOK TIME: 25 MINS | SERVES: 5

INGREDIENTS:

- 1 cup tri-color quinoa
  1½ cups water

- 1 tsp. onion powder

DIRECTIONS:

. Before starting, preheat the oven to 400°F.

. In a blender, all ingredients. Blend until smooth with no lumps.

. Line a baking pan with parchment paper (make sure the pan has a small lip).

. Evenly spread the quinoa blend on the baking sheet and put in the oven for 20-25 minutes.

. Remove from oven and allow to cool.

. Lift the bread out of the pan using the parchment paper and carefully peel bread from paper.

Quick tip: This is delicious as a sandwich or with a curry!

SPICY HOMEMADE TORTILLA CHIPS

COOK TIME: 16 MINS | SERVES: 6

INGREDIENTS:

- 12 corn tortillas
  1 tsp. olive oil
- ¼ tsp. chili powder
- ¼ tsp. cumin powder

- ¼ tsp. garlic powder
- ¼ tsp. paprika powder
- Himalayan sea salt

DIRECTIONS:

. Before starting, preheat the oven to 425°F. Line 2 large baking pans with parchment paper.

. Slice each tortilla into 6 triangles, then place on the baking pans, trying not to overlap. Place in oven and cook for 10 minutes.

. Take the baking pans out of the oven and delicately brush oil over the surface side of the chips (use only a little, otherwise the chips won't be crispy)

. Mix the spices and salt together and sprinkle over the chips.

. Put the chips back in the oven for another 6 minutes, or until crispy and golden.

HEALTHY CEREAL BARS

COOK TIME: 30 MINS | SERVES: 9

INGREDIENTS:

- ½ cup toasted almonds
- 1 ½ cup oats
- ½ cup almond flour
- ½ cup pure maple syrup
- ½ cup raisins
- ¼ cup almond butter
- 2 tablespoons chia seeds
- 1 tbsp. fractionated coconut oil
- 1 tsp. vanilla extract

- ½ tsp. cinnamon powder
- ¼ tsp. Himalayan pink sea salt
- 1/8 tsp. nutmeg powder

DIRECTIONS:

1. Go ahead and preheat oven to 325°F.

2. Use an 8x8 inch baking tin and grease and line with non-stick parchment paper.

3. Slice the almonds and add to a large bowl alongside the oats, almond flour, syrup, raisins, almond butter, chia seeds, oil, vanilla, cinnamon, salt, and nutmeg. Mix until it all sticks together.

4. Pat the almond mix into the pan, making sure the top is even. Put in the oven for 25 to 30 minutes, or until the edges of the pan are golden.

5. Allow to cool completely before cutting into even squares. Store in an airtight container.

BLACK BEAN TAQUITOS

COOK TIME: 20 MINS | SERVES: 12

INGREDIENTS:

- Olive oil
- 1 onion
- 1 poblano chile pepper
- 1 jalapeño chile pepper
- 4 garlic cloves
- 1 can black beans
- ½ cup cilantro leaves

- 1 tsp. chili powder
- 1 tsp. cumin powder
- 1 tsp. sea salt
- 24 corn tortillas

DIRECTIONS:

- Preheat your oven to 400°F.
- Use a large baking pan and line it with parchment paper then grease with oil.
- Chop your onion into quarters. Half both peppers and deseed them before chopping into quarters.
- Using a food processor, add onion, poblano pepper, jalapeño pepper, and garlic. Use the chopping blade and pulse 3 times before adding the black beans, cilantro, chili powder, cumin, and salt.
- Pulse another 3 times or until the mixture is finely chopped (you can pulse more if you want a smoother mix).
- Put the tortillas on a pan and heat them in the oven for about a minute, or until soft and pliable.
- Smear a large tablespoon of bean mix across each tortilla. Tightly roll like a burrito with open edges and put on a baking pan with the edge facing down. Leave a smidge of space between each tortilla and cook for 20 minutes or until golden.

Quick tip: These are great with dips like queso or salsa!

VEGETABLE TACOS

COOK TIME: 35 MINS | SERVES: 6

INGREDIENTS:

- 1 head of cauliflower
- 1 sweet potato
- 1 onion
- 2 tbsp. olive oil
- 1/8 tsp. Himalayan sea salt
- 1/8 tsp. black pepper
- 1 can chickpeas
- ½ cup BBQ

DIRECTIONS:

1. Preheat your oven to 425°F and put a sheet of parchment paper on a large baking tray.
2. Chop the cauliflower into small florets, the sweet potato into inch sized cubes, and dice the onion into small pieces.
3. Evenly place the cauliflower, sweet potato, and onion across the baking tray. Sprinkle oil, salt, and peppe across and mix to coat. Put in the oven for 10 to 15 minutes.
4. Take the tray out of the oven and dump the chickpeas on top. Pour ½ cup of BBQ sauce on top and stir to coat. Bake for another 8 minutes, or until the vegetable are soft.

Quick tip: This is great with any kind of taco, but especially on a corn tortilla with avocado, cilantro, coleslaw, and tomatoes!

SAVORY SWEET POTATOES

COOK TIME: 35 MINS | SERVES: 2

INGREDIENTS:

2 sweet potatoes
- 1 tsp. garlic powder
- 1/2 tsp. cumin powder
1/2 tsp. chili powder
- 1/2 tsp. Himalayan sea salt
1/2 tsp. black pepper

DIRECTIONS:

. Before starting, preheat your oven to 425°F.

. Peel the sweet potatoes and quarter lengthwise.

. In a pot, put a couple inches of water and bring to a boil. Put a steamer tray on top of the pot (make sure it is above the water) and put the potato pieces in the steamer. Put a lid on and steam for 7 minutes or until the potatoes have just become soft.

. Put a sheet of parchment paper on a large baking pan before moving the potatoes onto the pan. Make sure there is a bit of space between each piece

. Whisk together the garlic, cumin, chili, salt, and pepper. Evenly powder over the potato pieces.

. Put the tray in the oven for 10 minutes, then turn all the pieces and cook for another 10 minutes.

. Serve!

WINTER GREENS

COOK TIME: 1 HR 20 MINS | SERVES: 6

INGREDIENTS:

- 1/2 can chickpeas
- 1 cup scallions
- 4 garlic cloves
- 1 cup kale
- 1 1/3 cups dandelion leaves
- 3 cups spinach
- ¾ cup Swiss chard
- 1 tsp. jalapeño

- 2/3 cup bunch dill
- ¼ tsp. ground cloves
- ¼ tsp. cinnamon powder
- 1 tsp. lemon juice
- Himalayan sea salt

DIRECTIONS:

1. Finely chop the scallions, garlic, kale, dandelion, spinach, swiss chard, and jalapeñ0. Destem the dill and finely chop.

2. Put the chickpeas in a pot with 1 cup of water and bring to a boil before reducing heat to a simmer. Leave with a lid halfway on for 30-45 minutes until tender. Drain the water and set the chickpeas aside.

3. In a large pot, add the scallions, garlic, and ½ cup of water. Cover and simmer over medium heat for 10 minutes.

4. In the pot with the scallions, add all the greens, jalapeño, cloves, cinnamon, lemon juice, pinch of salt, and another cup of water. Keep at a simmer for another 10 minutes and stir every so often.

5. Transfer the greens to a blender and pulse until a chunky puree, but not so much it becomes a sauce.

6. Put the blended greens back into the pot and add the chickpeas. Stir over medium heat for another 5 minutes.

7. Serve hot!

LETTUCE BEAN BURRITOS

COOK TIME: 5 MINS | SERVES: 4

INGREDIENTS:

- 1 can white beans
- Head of romaine lettuce
- 1 red onion
- 1/2 cup basil
- 1 organic tomato
- 2 tbsp. lemon juice

- Himalayan pink salt
- Black pepper

DIRECTIONS:

Rinse and drain the beans.

Pull off 8 of the largest lettuce leaves and chop the hard stem off the bottom and set aside. Finely chop the onion and basil. Core and dice the tomato.

Mix together the beans, onion, tomato, basil, lemon juice, and a pinch of salt and pepper.

To shape the wraps, spread a spoonful of the white bean mix down the middle of each lettuce leaf and roll the leaf like a burrito.

Place seam-side down on a platter and serve.

MANGO CHUTNEY WRAPS

COOK TIME: 8 MINS | SERVES: 8

INGREDIENTS:

- 3 ripe mangoes
- 1 avocado
- 4 tbsp. lime juice
- 2 tbsp. coconut oil
- 2 tbsp. tahini
- 1 tsp. chili flakes
- ½ cup coriander leaves
- Sea salt

- 1 tbsp. fresh ginger
- 16 sheets of rice paper
- 3 carrots
- 2 bell peppers
- 1 cucumber
- Black pepper

DIRECTIONS:

1. Peel the skin off the mangos and cut the mango meat off the pit, keeping one mango flesh separate. Cut the avocado in half, remove the pit, and scoop out the flesh.

2. Add the mango flesh of 2 mangos to a blender along with the avocado, 2 tbsp. lime juice, oil, tahini, chili, coriander leaves, and a pinch of salt.

3. Peel the skin off the ginger and roughly chop before adding to the blender. Pulse then blend until smooth.

4. Pour the blended mango into a bowl and refrigerate until serving.

5. Chop the remaining mango flesh into slices.

6. To prepare the wraps, carefully dip the rice paper into hot water for no more than 10 seconds, then lay them flat and let dry for 2 minutes.

7. While you wait, thinly slice your carrots, peppers, and cucumber.

8. After the wraps have dried, spread a tbsp. of mango dip down the middle of each sheet of rice paper. Put the dried mango slices and vegetable slices in the middle. Dribble some lime juice on top and a smidge of salt and pepper, then roll up like a burrito.

9. Serve with more mango dip on the side!

Quick Tip: If you don't have access to rice paper, try using sushi seaweed strips for a twist! Instead of dipping it in water, just lightly brush some across.

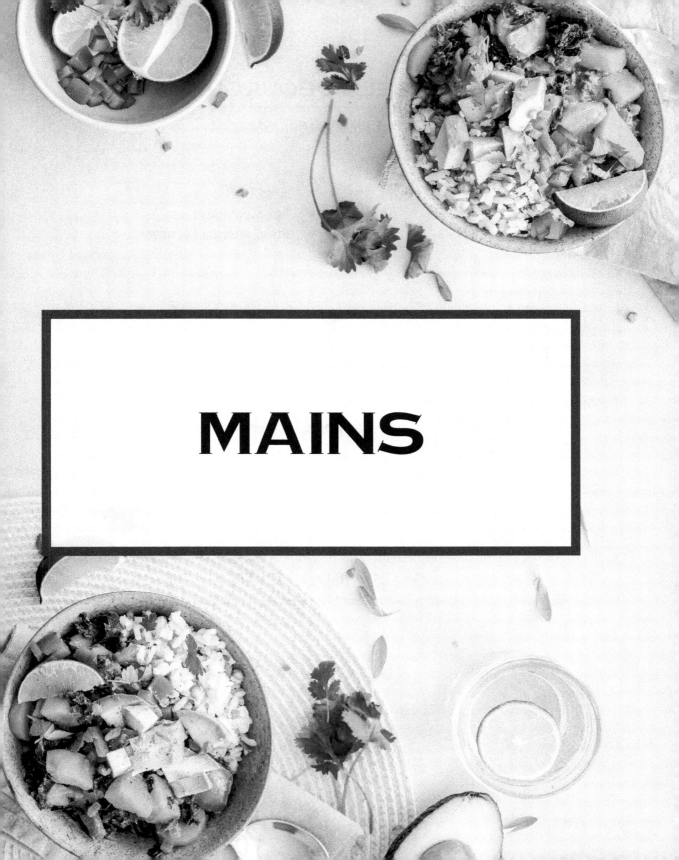

MAINS

PORTABELLA BOURGUIGNON

COOK TIME: 65 MINS | SERVES: 4

INGREDIENTS:

- 2 (8oz) packets portabella mushrooms
- 2 yellow onions
- 2 russet potatoes
- 3 carrots
- 3 garlic cloves
- 2 tbsp. tomato paste
- 1 cup dry red wine
- 1 bay leaf

- ¼ tsp. black pepper
- 1 tbsp. light soy sauce
- 1 tbsp. arrowroot powder

DIRECTIONS:

1. Preheat oven to 400°F.

2. Wash the mushrooms before carefully slicing them. Roughly chop the onions, potatoes, and carrots. Finely chop the garlic.

3. Line a baking tray with parchment paper and lay out the mushrooms on top. Put in the oven and bake for 20 minutes.

4. While waiting on the mushrooms, cook the onions in a little bit of water in a pan over medium high heat until translucent.

5. In a large pot over medium heat, combine all ingredients (excluding the arrowroot powder) Add 2 cups of water, then cover with a lid. Turn the heat down and simmer for 45 minutes.

6. After 45 minutes, add arrowroot powder. Stir to incorporate it and serve.

BLACK BEAN BURGERS

COOK TIME: 40 MINS | SERVES: 6

INGREDIENTS:

- 1 red onion
- 2 carrots
- 4 garlic cloves
- 1 can black beans
- ½ cup fresh parsley
- ¼ cup sun-dried tomatoes
- 1 cup oats
- 4 tbsp. olive oil

- ½ cup toasted pumpkin
- 1 tsp. cumin powder
- 1 tsp. paprika
- 1 tsp. chili powder
- ¾ tsp. salt
- ¼ tsp. black pepper
- ¼ tsp. red pepper flakes

DIRECTIONS:

Finely dice onion and shred carrots. Cut the garlic cloves in half. Drain and rinse the beans. Remove the parsley leaves from the stem. Drain and chop the tomatoes.

Using a strong blender or food processor, pulse until the oats are chopped coarsely. Leave oats in the food processor for later.

In a pan over medium high heat, add 1 tbsp. oil. Once the oil is hot, add the onion and carrots. Cook for 10 minutes. Combine with the garlic and stir for another 30 seconds.

Combine the onion with the oats in the food processor. Also add the beans, parsley, pumpkin seeds, tomatoes, cumin, paprika, chili powder, salt, and both peppers. Repeatedly pulse until all ingredients are chopped finely. The mixture should stick together, but not be pureed.

Using parchment paper, line a baking pan. Scoop the mixture into 6 even balls, then flatten into a burger shape. Cover the pan with a cloth and put them in the fridge until they are firm to the touch.

In a pan over medium high heat, add a couple tbsp. of oil. Once the oil is hot, set each patty in the pan, leaving a little space between each one. Cook on one side for 8 minutes, then flip and cook for another 8 minutes. The bean burgers are done when they are hot all the way through and browned on the edges.

Quick tip: Serve on burger buns or a bed of lettuce with toppings such as avocado, sprouts, and other veggies.

VEGAN GLUTEN-FREE PIZZA

COOK TIME: 50 MINS | SERVES: 2

INGREDIENTS:

- 1½ cups quinoa
- 2 tsp. Italian pizza seasoning
- 2 garlic cloves
- Himalayan pink salt
- 1/3 cup olive oil
- ¾ cup pesto
- ½ cup bulb of fennel
- ¼ cup red onion

- 1 cup arugula
- Black pepper

DIRECTIONS:

1. The night before, soak the quinoa in 6 cups of water overnight.

2. When you are ready to start, preheat your oven to 450°F.

3. Drain and rinse the quinoa from the day before. Put it into a blender or food processor with ¼ cup of water, seasoning, garlic, and 1 tsp. salt. Blend until the ingredients become a puree (if needed, add more water to make it thick but smooth).

4. Use a heat-proof pan with a lip and warm it in the oven for 5 minutes. Add ¼ cup oil and heat again for 5 minutes. Remove and swirl to make sure the oil coats the pan's surface.

5. Pour the quinoa batter into the pan and make sure to spread evenly. Return to the oven for 15 minutes or until the top is crispy.

6. Remove from the oven and use a spatula to flip the crust over like a large pancake. Bake for 10 more minutes.

7. Move the crust to a cooling rack and dab with a paper towel to remove extra oil. Repeat the process with the pan, but leave just a little bit in.

8. Thinly slice your fennel and red onion.

9. Put the crust into the pan again, then smooth pesto on top. Sprinkle the fennel and onion on top and bake for another 10-15 minutes.

10. Mix the arugula with 1 tsp. oil and a pinch of salt and pepper. Evenly spread over the pizza and serve promptly.

DELICIOUS VEGAN TACOS

COOK TIME: 20 MINS | SERVES: 6

INGREDIENTS:

- 2 tbsp. lime juice
- 2 tbsp. taco seasoning
- 1 tsp. honey
- 3 tbsp. olive oil
- 1 sweet potato
- 4 poblano chile peppers
- 1 red onion

- 2 portobello mushrooms
- Himalayan pink salt
- Black pepper
- 12 corn tortillas

DIRECTIONS:

Go ahead and preheat your oven to 450°F. You will be using a baking tray with a lip. Put it in the oven now to get it warm.

Whisk together the lime juice, seasoning, honey, and 2 tbsp. olive oil.

In a small bowl, combine the lime juice, taco seasoning, maple syrup, and 2 tablespoons oil and stir well.

Cut the sweet potato into stripes. Seed and cut the peppers. Peel the onion, cut it in half, then slice it thinly. Cut the mushrooms into thick slices.

In a bowl, add together the sweet potato, peppers, and onion. Add the lime sauce and stir to evenly coat everything. Mix in the mushrooms and stir to coat.

Using the pan from the oven, pour a dash of oil into it and swirl to cover the surface. Evenly spread the veggies across the pan and sprinkle with a pinch of salt and pepper. Cook for 20 minutes or until the potato is softened.

Serve by warming the tortillas in the microwave, then scooping the veggies into the tortilla. Add your favorite toppings and enjoy!

Quick tip: These are absolutely scrumptious with avocado and cilantro!

VEGAN POT PIE

COOK TIME: 1 HR 35 MINS | SERVES: 6

INGREDIENTS:

- 4 russet potatoes
- 2 yellow onions
- 3 carrots
- 4 heads of broccoli
- Sea salt
- 3 cups canned peas
- 3 cups canned corn

- 6 tablespoons arrowroot powder
- 4 cups almond milk
- ¼ cup nutritional yeast
- Black pepper

DIRECTIONS:

1. Peel the potatoes and cut them into large chunks. Finely dice the onions and carrots. Chop the broccoli florets from the stem.

2. Preheat your oven to 350°F.

3. Put the potatoes in a pot and cover with water. Bring the water to a boil, then turn down the heat, put on a lid, and cook for 14 minutes, or until the potatoes can be easily pierced.

4. Once the potatoes are soft, drain all the water except for 2/3 a cup. Move the potatoes and reserved water to a large bowl, then add ½ tbsp. of salt. Mash the potatoes using an electric mixer or hand masher.

5. Over medium-high heat, cook the onions and carrots on the stove. Stir constantly to prevent the veggies from sticking. Cook until the onions begin to brown, or about 8 minutes.

6. Add the broccoli, peas, and corn. Cook for another 6 minutes or until the broccoli can be easily pierced.

7. In another bowl, whisk together the arrowroot powder and almond milk. Add it to the cooking veggies. Also add the nutritional yeast and a sprinkle of salt and pepper. Cook for another 5 minutes or until it begins to thicken.

8. Pour the veggies into a 9 x 13-inch baking dish and evenly spread the mashed potatoes on top.

9. Cook in the oven for an hour, or until the top is slightly golden.

FILLING SQUASH BOWLS

COOK TIME: 45 MINS | SERVES: 2

INGREDIENTS:

- 1 spaghetti squash
- Sea salt
- Ground black pepper
- Dried oregano
- Dried basil
- Dried fennel
- 2 roasted red peppers
- 2 cups spinach
- ½ cup canned artichoke hearts

- ¼ cup Kalamata olives
- 1 tbsp. fresh basil
- ¼ cup sun-dried tomatoes
- 1 cup canned chickpeas
- 1 cup marinara

DIRECTIONS:

1. Preheat your oven to 400°F and use parchment paper to line a large baking tray.

2. Cut the squash into halves. Use a strong spoon to scoop out all the seeds. Season the squash according to your tastes with salt, pepper, and the herbs. Place each half cut-side down on the prepared tray and bake for 30 minutes. The squash should be soft all the way through.

3. Roughly chop the peppers, spinach, artichoke, olives, basil, and tomatoes. Combine all chopped ingredients except basil in a bowl with the chickpeas.

4. Prepare the squash by evenly spreading half of the pasta sauce into the squash. Divide the veggies evenly and fill each squash half. Pour remaining sauce on top and bake for 15 minutes.

5. Sprinkle with fresh basil and serve.

VEGAN ENCHILADAS

COOK TIME: 30 MINS | SERVES: 4

INGREDIENTS:

- 1 tsp. avocado oil
- 1 yellow onion
- 1 bunch kale
- 1 ripe avocado
- Black olives
- Fresh cilantro
- 2 cans pinto beans
- 2 teaspoons taco seasoning
- Sea salt

- Ground black pepper
- 1 jar salsa
- 12 wheat tortillas
- ½ cup dairy-free queso

DIRECTIONS:

1. Preheat your oven to 400°F and grease a 9 × 13-inch pan with the oil.

2. Dice the onion. Destem and chop the kale. Dice avocado, slice the olives, and chop the cilantro. Set aside the avocado, olives, and cilantro for later.

3. Drain and rinse the beans.

4. In the pan, add in layers the onion, kale, and beans. Sprinkle the taco seasoning over it along with a pinch of salt and pepper. Use half the salsa as the next layer, then use the tortillas for the next layer. Evenly spread the second half of the salsa on top of the tortillas and finish it off with the queso.

5. Cover the pan with tin foil and cook for 30 minutes. The veggies should be soft.

6. Before serving, let the pan cool for a few minutes. Serve with the avocado, olives, and a sprinkle of cilantro.

WARMING WINTER BEETS

COOK TIME: 1 HR 20 MINS | SERVES: 4

INGREDIENTS:

- 6 beetroots
- 2 cups buckwheat
- 3 tbsp. lemon juice
- 1 can coconut milk
- Sea salt
- Black pepper

DIRECTIONS:

1. Preheat the oven to 410°F.
2. Put the beets on a baking tray and put them into the oven for an hour. No need to peel or cut. After an hour, they should be soft and the skin crisp. Remove from oven and let cool.
3. Rinse the buckwheat until the water runs clear, then put in a pot with 3 ½ cups of water. Bring to a boil, then reduce the heat and simmer for 15 minutes. The water should have all evaporated and the buckwheat should be a little bit hard.
4. Peel the beets. The skin should come off easily. Put the peeled beets into a food processor. Add the lemon juice, coconut milk, and a pinch of salt and pepper. Blend until the beet mix is smooth.
5. Stir the beet mix into the buckwheat over medium heat. Stir for a couple minutes or until warmed through, then serve.

SAUTEED BOK CHOY

COOK TIME: 10 MINS | SERVES: 5

INGREDIENTS:

- 1½ lbs. bok choy
- 1 tbsp. fresh ginger
- 2 tbsp. light soy sauce
- 1 tsp. honey
- 2 tbsp. sesame oil

DIRECTIONS:

1. Cut the bok choy stems in half long-ways, then cut into ½ inch chunks. Cut the greens into similar sized pieces. Grate the ginger.
2. Mix together the soy sauce and honey until thoroughly combined.
3. Over high heat, warm the oil in a pan. Place in the cut bok choy stems and stir constantly for 5 minutes. Add the ginger and stir for 30 seconds. Add the bok choy greens and dressing. Stir often for at least 1 minute, or until the greens are cooked and wilted.

Quick tip: Serve over rice, and try adding tofu!

THREE BEAN CHILI

COOK TIME: 1 HR 20 MINS | SERVES: 8

INGREDIENTS:

- 1 tbsp. avocado oil
- 1 onion
- 1 bell pepper
- 2 jalapeño peppers
- 4 garlic cloves
- 1 can kidney beans
- 1 can pinto beans
- 1 can black beans
- 1 cup green onions
- ¼ cup fresh cilantro

- 2 avocados
- ¼ cup chili powder
- 1 tbsp. cumin powder
- 1 tbsp. cacao powder
- ¼ tsp. cinnamon powder
- 1 can tomato chunks
- 1 tbsp. honey
- Himalayan pink salt
- Black pepper

DIRECTIONS:

1. Finely dice the onion, bell pepper, and one jalapeño, making sure to remove the pepper seeds first. Mince the garlic. Drain and rinse all the beans. Thinly slice the green onions and remaining jalapeño. Chop the cilantro and dice the avocados.

2. In a large pot, add the oil and heat over medium-high. Toss in the onion and bell pepper. Stir for 10 minutes.

3. Add into the pot, the first jalapeño pepper and the garlic. Mix, then add the chili powder, cumin, cacao, and cinnamon. Stir constantly for 2 minutes.

4. Toss in the tomatoes, beans, and honey. If it becomes too thick, add a little water. Stir to combine. Lower the heat and allow to simmer for 45 minutes. Season to taste with salt and pepper.

5. To serve, top with the diced jalapeño, green onions, cilantro, and avocado.

SWEET POTATO NOODLES

COOK TIME: 30 MINS | SERVES: 4

INGREDIENTS:

- 1 small onion
- 2 garlic cloves
- 1-inch piece fresh ginger
- ¾ cup almond butter
- 1 tbsp. soy sauce
- 1 tbsp. lemon juice
- 1 tbsp. maple syrup
- 1 tsp. paprika

- ⅛ tsp. red pepper flakes
- Himalayan pink salt
- Black pepper
- ¼ cup water
- 2 sweet potatoes
- ¼ cup olive oil
- ½ cup green onions
- ½ cup fresh parsley

DIRECTIONS:

1. Preheat your oven to 425°F and use parchment paper to line a baking pan with a lip.

2. Roughly chop the onion, garlic, and ginger.

3. Add to a food processor the onion, ginger, and garlic. Use the chopping blade and pulse until the ingredients are finely chopped.

4. Add the almond butter, soy sauce, lemon juice, maple syrup, paprika, red pepper, and a pinch of salt and pepper. Pulse until thoroughly incorporated.

5. Put the blender on low and pour water through the hole in the lid. Keep blending until the mixture is creamy and smooth.

6. Use a tool to spiralize the sweet potatoes.

7. Put the potatoes in a bowl. Add the oil and toss to coat. Spread the potato noodles on the previously prepped baking pan. Sprinkle with salt and pepper.

8. Cook the potatoes for 20 minutes, but check regularly to make sure some noodles aren't cooking too fast. If some are, remove them and set aside.

9. While waiting on the noodles, chop green onions and parsley.

10. To serve, spoon the noodles and then top with the sauce, green onions, and parsley.

SPECIAL SPRING ROLLS

COOK TIME: 25 MINS | SERVES: 4

INGREDIENTS:

- 1 stalk celery
- ¼ cup shallots
- 1 tbsp. ginger root
- 4 garlic cloves
- 1 (8oz) packet button mushrooms
- 2 cups walnuts
- 1 cup shredded carrots
- ½ cup raw cashews
- 2 tbsp. fresh mint

- 1/3 cup fresh cilantro
- ¼ cup green onions
- 2 tbsp. olive oil
- 2 tbsp. lime juice
- 2 tbsp. soy sauce
- 2 tbsp. honey
- 1 tbsp. rice vinegar
- Red pepper flakes
- 12 leaves butter lettuce

DIRECTIONS:

1. To prep, thinly slice the celery. Mince the shallots, ginger, and garlic. Finely chop the mushrooms and walnuts. Shred the carrots and chop the cashews. Chop the mint and cilantro. Finely slice the green onions.

2. Set aside the carrots, cashews, green onions, and most of the cilantro.

3. Over medium-high heat, heat the oil in a large pan. Add the celery and shallots and stir for 5 minutes. Add the garlic and ginger and stir for another minute.

4. Add the mushrooms to the pan. Stir constantly until the mushrooms have dried a bit and begun to brown.

5. Add the walnuts and cook for a couple of minutes until they are toasted.

6. Add the lime juice, soy sauce, honey, and vinegar. Lower the heat and allow everything to come to a simmer for 15 minutes. The sauce should become a bit thicker.

7. Remove the pan from the heat and add the mint, 2 tbsp. cilantro, and pepper flakes.

8. Serve by spooning the mixture into the lettuce leaves and topping with carrots, cashews, green onions, and remaining cilantro.

SPICY VEGETABLE CURRY

COOK TIME: 30 MINS | SERVES: 4

INGREDIENTS:

- 2 bell peppers
- 1 jalapeño pepper
- 4 garlic cloves
- 1 tbsp. fresh ginger
- 2 cans of chickpeas
- 2 tbsp. olive oil
- 1½ tsp. sea salt
- ½ tsp. black pepper

- 1 tbsp. curry powder
- 1 can tomato chunks
- 1 can coconut milk

DIRECTIONS:

- Deseed the bell peppers and cut into inch long pieces. Deseed the jalapeño and mince. Also mince the garlic and ginger. Drain and rinse the chickpeas.
- Over medium-high heat, warm the oil in a large pot.
- Combine the bell peppers, salt, and black pepper in the pot. Cook for 6 minutes, or until the peppers begin to brown.
- Then add the jalapeño, garlic, ginger, and curry. Cook for another minute.
- Mix in the chickpeas, tomatoes and juice, and coconut milk. Turn the heat to high and bring the contents to a boil. Cover with a lid, lower the heat, and simmer for 20 minutes or until the peppers are nice and soft.

Quick Tip: This is best served over rice!

SWEET POTATO NACHOS

COOK TIME: 30 MINS | SERVES: 2

INGREDIENTS:

- 2 sweet potatoes
- 2 tbsp. olive oil
- ½ tsp. cumin powder
- ½ tsp. paprika powder
- ½ tsp. chili powder
- ½ tsp. garlic powder
- ½ tsp. Himalayan pink salt
- 1 can black beans
- 1 large tomato

- 1 jalapeño pepper
- ½ cup pitted black olives
- ¼ cup green onions
- ½ cup fresh cilantro
- ½ cup guacamole
- 1 tbsp. nutritional yeast

DIRECTIONS:

1. Preheat your oven to 450°F and use parchment paper to line a baking tray.

2. Thinly slice the potatoes into rounds and toss with oil. Spread the potatoes in as even a layer as possible on the tray.

3. Mix together the cumin, paprika, chili powder, garlic powder in a small bowl, then toss over the potatoes

4. Put the potato tray in the oven for 20 minutes. The potatoes should be soft enough to stab easily.

5. Drain and rinse the black beans. Dice the tomato and finely slice the jalapeño, olives, and green onions. Chop the cilantro and set it aside.

6. Take the tray out of the oven and cover with the beans, tomato, pepper, olives, and green onion. Cook another 7 minutes or until everything is warmed through.

7. Before serving, sprinkle with cilantro. Serve alongside guacamole and nutritional yeast.

CABBAGE CURRY AND CHICKPEAS

COOK TIME: 35 MINS | SERVES: 4

INGREDIENTS:

- 7 tbsp. olive oil
- 1 tbsp. curry powder
- 1½ tsp. honey
- 1 tsp. sea salt
- ¼ tsp. black pepper
- 1 head cabbage
- 2 garlic cloves
- 2 tsp. fresh ginger

- 2 cups cherry tomatoes
- ¼ cup fresh cilantro
- 2 cans chickpeas

DIRECTIONS:

Preheat the oven to 500°F.

Mix together ¼ cup of oil, 2 tsp. curry powder, honey, salt, and pepper.

Halve the cabbage, then cut each half into 4ths (you should have 8 slices).

Evenly layer the cabbage on a baking tray, then coat with the oil mix. Cover with aluminum foil and cook for 10 minutes. Then, take off the foil and coat in another 2 tbsp. oil. Cook again for 15 minutes (uncovered).

Mince the garlic and grate the ginger. Halve the tomatoes and chop the cilantro.

In a pan over medium-high heat, warm 1 tbsp. oil. Mix in the garlic, ginger, and 1 tsp. curry powder. Stir for a minute before adding the chickpeas, its liquid, and the tomatoes. Bring to a simmer for 8 minutes, stirring often. The mix should have thickened slightly.

To serve, plate the cabbage and scoop the veggies on top. Sprinkle with cilantro for an extra touch.

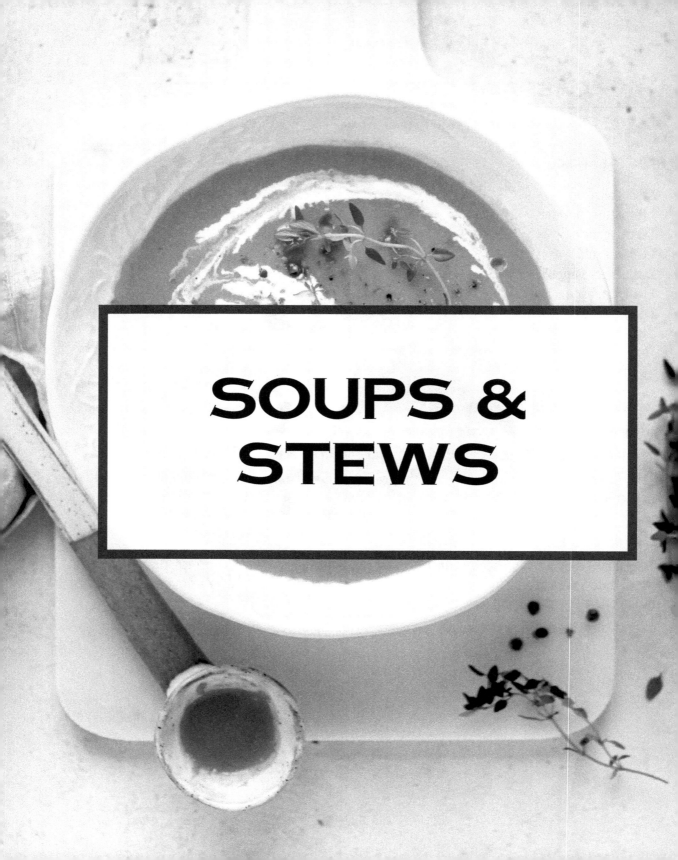

SOUPS & STEWS

MUSHROOM KALE STEW

COOK TIME: 1 HR 20 MINS | SERVES: 8

INGREDIENTS:

- 2 onions
- 3 garlic cloves
- 4 potatoes
- 2 (8oz) packets button mushrooms
- 1 bunch kale
- 1 bay leaf
- ½ tsp. dried dill
- 1 tsp. onion powder

- 4 cups vegetable stock
- 2 cups non-dairy milk
- ¼ cup nutritional yeast
- 1 tbsp. soy sauce

DIRECTIONS:

1. Preheat the oven to 400°F.

2. Finely dice the onions. Mince the garlic. Chop the potatoes into cubes. Slice the mushrooms. Finely chop the kale.

3. Line a baking tray with parchment paper and place the mushrooms on it. Put in the oven for 30 minutes.

4. While waiting on the mushrooms, put 3 tbsp. of water in a pot and heat up over medium heat.

5. Add the onions to the pot and stir for 5 minutes before adding all the spices and cooking another 5 minutes.

6. Mix in the kale, potatoes, vegetable stock, and cooked mushrooms. Cook for another 30 minutes.

7. Now add the milk, nutritional yeast, and soy sauce.

8. Scoop out 2 cups of the soup and use a blender to blend it into a puree. Mix it back into the pot and stir to mix.

9. Serve hot.

TOMATO HERB SOUP

COOK TIME: 35 MINS | SERVES: 8

INGREDIENTS:

- 16 tomatoes
- 4 bell peppers
- 4 tbsp. herbes de Provence
- Sea salt
- Black pepper
- Avocado oil
- ½ cup basil
- 1 can white kidney beans

- 4 tbsp. tomato paste
- 4 cups vegetable broth
- 2 tbsp. soy sauce

DIRECTIONS:

1. Preheat your oven to 375°F.
2. Chop the tomatoes into four pieces. Deseed the peppers before slicing into thick strips.
3. Prepare a baking sheet with parchment paper, then put the tomatoes and peppers on it along with the herbs, salt, and pepper.
4. Place these on a baking tray with the herbes de Provence, salt, and pepper. Coat all of it in oil and cook for 30 minutes.
5. Use a strong blender to puree the cooked tomato and pepper with the basil, beans, tomato paste, broth, and soy sauce. Blend until smooth.
6. Move the pureed soup to a pot and heat through before serving.

BEAN PEA SOUP

COOK TIME: 15 MINS | SERVES: 5

INGREDIENTS:

- 5 cups peas
- 3 1/3 cups vegetable broth
- 1 can white kidney beans
- 1/4 cup mint leaves
- Sea salt
- Black pepper

DIRECTIONS:

Over medium-high heat, warm the peas in a large pot until they begin to boil (roughly 10 minutes).

Using a blender, puree the peas, broth, beans, and mint until smooth.

Transfer the blended soup back to the pot and heat through. Add a pinch of salt and pepper, mix well, then serve.

Quick tip: This soup is also delicious chilled!

SPINACH BEAN SOUP

COOK TIME: 40 MINS | SERVES: 8

INGREDIENTS:

- 2 yellow onions
- 2 garlic cloves
- 2 russet potatoes
- 1 can coconut milk
- 1 can tomato puree
- 2 cans white kidney beans
- 4 cups water
- 1 tsp. turmeric powder
- 1 tsp. black pepper
- 2 tsp. dried lime
- 1 tsp. soy sauce
- 6 cups of spinach

DIRECTIONS:

Roughly chop the onions and mince the garlic. Dice the potatoes.

In a pot over medium-high heat, warm 4 tbsp. of water. Add the onions and cook for 5 minutes, or until they begin to turn translucent.

Mix in all the remaining ingredients, save the spinach. Turn the heat down slightly and let simmer for 10 minutes.

Incorporate the spinach, stir, and let simmer for another 25 minutes before serving.

THICK CAULIFLOWER RICE SOUP

COOK TIME: 50 MINS | SERVES: 8

INGREDIENTS:

- 1½ cups brown rice
- 1 head of cauliflower
- 1 yellow onion
- 3 carrots
- 3 celery stalks
- 3 garlic cloves
- 1 tsp. dried oregano
- ½ tsp. dried thyme
- ½ tsp. black pepper
- ¼ tsp. sea salt
- 4¼ cups vegetable broth
- 4¼ cups water
- 3 tbsp. lemon juice
- ½ cup nutritional yeast

DIRECTIONS:

1. Prepare the rice according to the package.
2. Chop the stem from the cauliflower so you are left with bite-sized florets. Dice the onion, carrots, and celery. Mince the garlic.
3. Over medium-high heat, cook the onions until translucent, or about 5 minutes.
4. Mix in the carrots, celery, and garlic. Cook for 3 minutes.
5. Mix in the spices, cauliflower, vegetable broth, water, and lemon juice. Cook for 35 minutes over medium-high heat.
6. Check to make sure the cauliflower is soft before mixing in the nutritional yeast.
7. Transfer the contents of the pot to a blender and blend until smooth.
8. Move the blended soup back to the pot so it can warm through. Add the rice, mix, and serve.

THAI CURRY STEW

COOK TIME: 8 HRS | SERVES: 8

INGREDIENTS:

- 3 cups long-grain rice
- 1 yellow onion
- 2 carrots
- 2 golden potatoes
- 2 heads cauliflower
- 1 bunch kale
- 2 cups lentils
- 1 tbsp. olive oil

- ¼ cup Thai curry paste
- 1 can coconut milk
- 8 cups vegetable broth
- Sea salt

DIRECTIONS:

1. Cook the rice according to the package.

2. Dice the onion and the carrots. Chop the potatoes into chunks. Cup the cauliflower florets from the stem. Destem the kale and chop roughly. Rinse and drain the lentils.

3. Over medium-high heat, warm oil in a pan. Once the oil is hot, add the onion and cook until translucent (roughly 5 minutes).

4. Mix the curry paste in with the onions and keep stirring for 2 minutes.

5. Pour the coconut milk into the pan, then lower the heat and allow to slow contents to simmer for a couple minutes.

6. Use a large slow-cooker and add in the lentils, carrots, cauliflower, and potatoes. Add 6 cups of broth and the cooked onions. Make sure to stir before covering and cooking for 8 hours on low or 4 hours on high.

7. 30 minutes before the stew is done cooking, mix in the kale. If needed, add more broth. Also add a pinch of salt.

8. Serve with rice.

COCONUT CURRY

COOK TIME: 30 MINS | SERVES: 4

INGREDIENTS:

- 4 carrots
- 1 cup button mushrooms
- 2 zucchinis
- 4 cans coconut milk
- 4 tbsp. Thai curry paste
- 2 tsp. honey
- ½ tsp. sea salt

- ½ cup cashews
- ¼ cup green onions
- 1 chili pepper
- 1 lime

DIRECTIONS:

1. Thinly slice the carrots and mushrooms. Spiralize the zucchini.

2. Over medium high-heat, mix the coconut milk and curry paste in a pot. Bring to a simmer before mixing in the honey and salt.

3. Add the carrots and mushrooms, then cover and simmer for 20 minutes. The carrots should be soft enough to pierce.

4. Add the spiralized zucchini.

5. Chop the cashews, thinly slice the green onions and chili pepper. Cut the lime into wedges.

6. Serve with a sprinkle of cashews, green onions, and chili pepper. Place lime wedges on the side and enjoy!

VEGETABLE FAJITA SOUP

COOK TIME: 30 MINS | SERVES: 6

INGREDIENTS:

- 1 yellow onion
- 1 bell pepper
- 1 zucchini
- 4 garlic cloves
- 1 can black beans
- 1 can pinto beans
- ¾ cup fresh cilantro
- 1 tbsp. olive oil
- 2 tbsp. taco spice mix
- 4 cups vegetable broth

- 1 can tomato chunks
- 1 can chopped green chilies
- 1 cup frozen corn
- 2 tbsp. lime juice
- Himalayan pink salt
- Black pepper
- 3 soft avocados
- 1 lime
- 1 bag tortilla chips

DIRECTIONS:

1. Dice the onion, bell pepper, and zucchini. Mince the garlic. Drain and rinse all the beans. Pull the cilantro leaves from the stem and chop.

2. Over medium-high heat, warm the oil in a large pot before adding the onion and bell pepper. Stir for 5 minutes. The onions should look translucent.

3. Mix in the zucchini and garlic, stirring for another minute. Mix in the taco spices and stir for another minute or so to incorporate.

4. Pour in the broth and add the beans, tomatoes, and chilies. Mix well and bring to a boil. Turn down the heat and allow to simmer for 20 minutes.

5. Mix in the corn, lime juice, and ¼ cup cilantro. Add a pinch of salt and pepper. Mix well, then turn off heat.

6. Dice the avocados and slice the limes.

7. Serve by spooning into bowls. Garnish with tortilla chips, avocado, remaining cilantro, and a slice of lime.

SPICY CHICKPEA SOUP

COOK TIME: 40 MINS | SERVES: 4

INGREDIENTS:

- 1 cup chickpea flour
- 1 onion
- 1 tbsp. olive oil
- 2 tbsp. chili paste
- 2 cups water
- 1 can tomato chunks

DIRECTIONS:

1. Soak the flour in water overnight.
2. Peel and dice the onion.
3. In a large pot, heat oil over medium-heat. Add the chili paste and stir for a minute before adding the onion and cooking for another 3 minutes.
4. Mix in the water, flour, and can of tomatoes plus juice. Mix thoroughly then cover the pot with a lid and let simmer for 30 minutes. Stir every so often.
5. Place a medium stockpot over medium heat. Add oil and the spice blend and cook until fragrant, about 1 minute. Add the onion and cook until beginning to soften, about 3 minutes.
6. Add the water and flour, then the tomatoes with their juice. Stir to combine, cover, and cook for 30 minutes, stirring every 10 minutes.
7. Let cool before serving.

CABBAGE QUINOA STEW

COOK TIME: 30 MINS | SERVES: 6

INGREDIENTS:

- 4 carrots
- 1 large yellow onion
- 1 bunch bok choy
- 1 cup red cabbage
- 1 bell pepper
- 3 green onions
- 4 garlic cloves
- 1 oz dried shiitake mushrooms
- ½ cup red quinoa

- 1 tbsp. olive oil
- 2 tsp. turmeric powder
- 3 cups water
- 2 cups vegetable broth
- ¼ tsp. ground black pepper
- ¼ cup gluten-free red miso

DIRECTIONS:

1. Peel and slice the carrots into rounds. Chop the onion and bok choy. Finely chop the red cabbage and bell pepper. Thinly slice the green onions. Mince the garlic. Roughly chop or break up the mushrooms. Rinse and drain the quinoa.

2. Over medium-high heat, warm the oil in a large pot. Add in the carrots and onion. Stir for 5 minutes or until the carrots begin to soften.

3. Mix in the mushrooms, turmeric, and garlic. Stir, then mix in the water, broth, quinoa, and pepper.

4. Cover the pot and let simmer for 15 minutes.

5. After 15 minutes, mix in the bok choy and cabbage. Lower the heat slightly and cook for 3 minutes.

6. Mix the miso in with a whisk and then take off heat.

7. Just before serving, add the bell pepper and green onions. Spoon into bowls and serve.

TOFU MUSHROOM SOUP

COOK TIME: 40 MINS | SERVES: 6

INGREDIENTS:

- 1 package extra-firm tofu
- 6 green onions
- 1 inch piece fresh ginger
- 4 garlic cloves
- 1 package shiitake mushrooms
- ¼ cup dried porcini mushrooms
- 3 cups watercress
- 1 tbsp. olive oil

- ¼ cup cooking sherry
- 4 cups vegetable broth
- 2 tbsp. light soy sauce

DIRECTIONS:

1. Wrap the tofu in paper towels and then set a weight on top. Let it sit for 20 minutes, then cut it into bite-sized pieces.

2. Separate the white and green parts of the green onions and mince the white part. Thinly slice the green part.

3. Grate the ginger and mince the garlic. Destem the shiitake mushrooms and cut into slices. Mince the porcini mushrooms. Remove the stems from the watercress.

4. Over medium heat, warm the oil in a large pot before adding the whites of the green onions, ginger, and garlic. Stir for a minute.

5. Mix in both kinds of mushrooms, then cover for 5 minutes or until the mushrooms are softer.

6. Mix in the sherry and simmer for a minute, or until mostly evaporated.

7. Mix in the broth and leave uncovered to simmer for 10 minutes.

8. Mix in the watercress, soy sauce, and tofu chunks. Simmer for 5 minutes.

9. Add the green part of the green onions and a pinch of pepper. Add a little more soy sauce if desired and serve.

SOUTH EAST ASIAN SOUP

COOK TIME: 45 MINS | SERVES: 8

INGREDIENTS:

- 1 package firm tofu
- 1 package shiitake mushrooms
- 2 stalks lemongrass
- 2 tbsp. fresh ginger
- 1 garlic clove
- 6oz snow peas
- 3 green onions
- 1 tbsp. olive oil
- 4 tsp. red curry paste

- 6 cups vegetable broth
- 3 tbsp. soy sauce
- 1 tbsp. honey
- 2 cans coconut milk
- 3 tbsp. lime juice
- Sea salt
- Black pepper
- ½ cup fresh cilantro

DIRECTIONS:

1. Wrap the tofu in paper towels and then set a weight on top. Let it sit for 20 minutes, then cut it into bite-sized pieces.

2. Destem the mushrooms and cut into chunks. Mince the bottom 6 inches of the lemongrass and mince. Also mince the ginger and garlic. Cut the peas into ½ inch pieces. Thinly slice the green parts of the green onions.

3. In a large pot over medium heat, warm the oil before adding the mushrooms, lemongrass, ginger, and garlic. Stir for 30 seconds, then mix in the curry paste. Stir for another 30 seconds.

4. Mix in ½ cup of broth to fully incorporate everything before adding the rest of the broth.

5. Mix in the soy sauce and honey. Bring everything to a boil then turn down the heat to low. Partially cover and allow to simmer for 20 minutes.

6. After 20 minutes, mix in the tofu, coconut milk, snow peas, lime juice, and a pinch of salt and pepper. Cook for 5 minutes or until the peas are softened.

7. To serve, spoon into bowls and garnish with cilantro leaves and green onion.

FIERY LENTIL SOUP

COOK TIME: 45 MINS | SERVES: 8

INGREDIENTS:

- ⅓ cup coconut oil
- 1 onion
- 2 celery stalks
- 1 tbsp. fresh ginger
- 5 garlic cloves
- ¾ cup fresh cilantro
- ½ cup fresh parsley
- 1 can chickpeas
- 1 cup lentils beans
- 4 ounces Swiss chard
- 2 tsp. coriander powder

- 2 tsp. paprika powder
- 1 tsp. cumin powder
- ½ tsp. cinnamon powder
- ⅛ tsp. red pepper flakes
- 8 cups vegetable broth
- 1 can tomato chunks
- ½ cup risoni pasta
- 2 tbsp. lemon juice
- Sea salt
- Black pepper

DIRECTIONS:

1. Finely chop the onion and celery. Mince the ginger, garlic, cilantro, and parsley. Rinse and drain the chick-peas. Rinse and drain the lentils. Destem the Swiss chard and cut into chunks.

2. In a large pot over medium-high heat, warm the oil before adding the onion and celery. Cook for about 8 minutes, or until the onion becomes translucent.

3. Turn the heat to medium and mix in the garlic and ginger. Cook for 1 minute, then add the coriander, paprika, cumin, cinnamon, and pepper flakes. Cook for 1 minute. Mix in ½ cup of cilantro and ¼ cup of parsley. Cook for 1 minute.

4. Pour in the broth, chickpeas, and lentils. Turn the heat to high and bring to a boil. Immediately reduce the heat to medium-low and partially cover with a lid. Allow to simmer for 20 minutes, or until the lentils are tender.

5. Mix in the tomatoes and pasta. Partially cover and simmer again for 7 minutes. Stir occasionally.

6. Mix in the Swiss chard and put the lid partially back on. Cook for another 5 minutes or until the pasta is soft.

7. Remove from heat and mix in the lemon juice, and remaining cilantro and parsley. Add a pinch of salt and pepper.

8. Make sure to mix thoroughly, then serve.

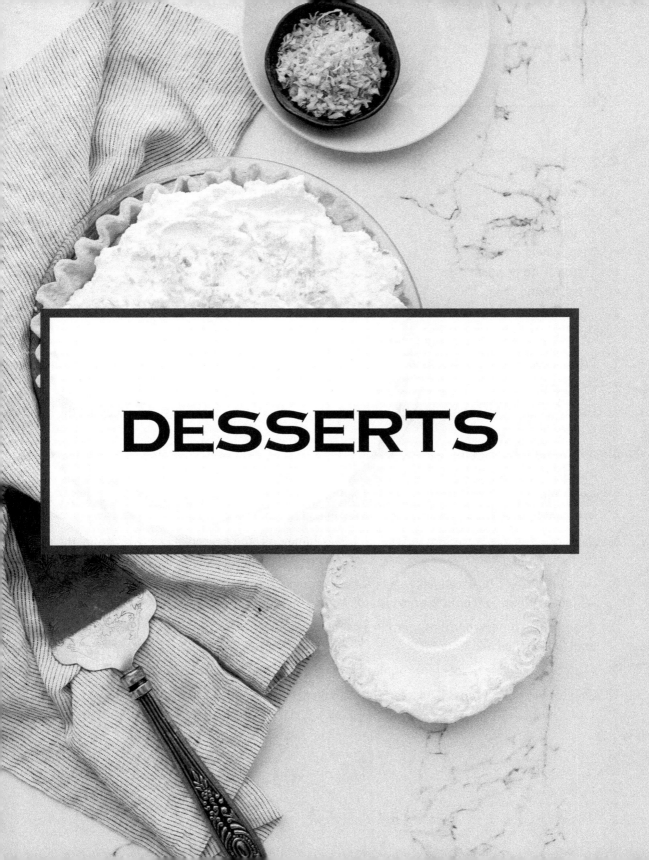

DESSERTS

3-LAYER COOKIE BARS

COOK TIME: 50 MINS | SERVES: 8

INGREDIENTS:

- 1 can chickpeas
- 1 cup honey
- 1 cup almond butter
- 2 tsp. vanilla extract
- 1 tsp. baking powder
- ½ tsp. baking soda

- Himalayan pink salt
- ¼ tsp. cinnamon powder
- ½ cup gluten-free oats
- 1 tbsp. fractionated coconut oil
- 1 bar dark vegan chocolate
- 2 tbsp. oat milk

DIRECTIONS:

1. Preheat your oven to 350°F. Prep a 9 × 9-inch baking pan by greasing it or inserting parchment paper.

2. Drain and rinse your chickpeas.

3. Use a food processor to mix together the chickpeas and 1/3 cup honey. Pulse until they are thick and buttery.

4. Add ½ cup almond butter, vanilla, baking powder, baking soda, ½ tsp. salt, and cinnamon. Pulse again until incorporated. Pour in the oats and keep pulsing until mostly smooth.

5. Scoop the batter into the baking pan and put in the oven for 20 minutes. They may look a little uncooked in the middle, but it will set as it cools. Leave in pan to cool.

6. Use a whisk to mix ½ cup almond butter, 1 tbsp. honey, oil, and a pinch of salt. Whisk until the mixture is smooth.

7. Once the baked bars have totally cooled, evenly spread the almond butter mixture on top. Chill in the refrigerator or freezer until the top is hard.

8. Use a double broiler (or a glass bowl in a pot of hot water) to melt the chocolate. Mix in the milk and stir until fully melted and smooth.

9. Allow the chocolate to cool for a couple of minutes, then evenly spread it in the pan.

10. Chill again until the top is hard, then slice into pieces. Store leftovers in the fridge.

PEACH DATE PIE

COOK TIME: 35 MINS | SERVES: 10

INGREDIENTS:

- 2 cups almond flour
- 1 cup dates
- 4 peaches
- 1 tsp. arrowroot powder

- 2 dates
- ¾ cups water

DIRECTIONS:

First, preheat your oven to 350°F.

In a food processor, combine the almond flour and 1 cup of dates. Blend until sticky.

Spoon the mixture into a cake pan and firmly press down to form a crust.

Cut the peaches in half and remove the pit. Set aside one half, then thinly slice the rest of them.

In a blender, add the half of the peach, the arrowroot powder, 2 dates, and the water. Pulse to blend. The mixture should become smooth.

Measure out 2/3rds of the blended mix and pour it into the crust.

Use the cut peach slices to make an even layer on top of the blend mix. For a fancy look, fan the slices from the edges to the middle.

Spread the rest of the blend mix on top and put in the oven for 35 minutes.

Let cool before slicing and serving.

COCONUT SCONES AND CREAM

COOK TIME: 30 MINS | SERVES: 6

INGREDIENTS:

- 2 cups oat flour
- 2 cups ground almonds
- 1 cup almond milk
- 4 tbsp. coconut sugar
- 3 tbsp. unsweetened applesauce
- 8 large strawberries
- ½ cup fresh blueberries
- 200g creamed coconut (this is different than coconut milk)
- strawberry jam

DIRECTIONS:

1. Preheat your oven to 360°F.
2. In a large bowl, mix together the coconut flour, ground almonds, milk, coconut sugar, and applesauce. The batter should be smooth.
3. Finely dice the strawberries, then mix into the batter. Add the blueberries and stir.
4. Cover two baking trays in parchment paper. Use a large spoon to scoop out batter and place on the pan i circles.
5. Put in the oven for 35–40 minutes. You should be able to know they're finished when the tops are golden.
6. Put the baked scones on a cooling rack while you make the cream.
7. Put the coconut cream package (don't open it) into a bowl of boiling water.
8. After the cream has melted, open it and put it into a new bowl with 3 tbsp. water. Use a stand or hand mixer to whisk until it is thick and creamy.
9. Serve by cutting open the scones and spreading them with coconut cream and the strawberry jam.

NO-COOK CHOC CHEESECAKE

COOK TIME: 2 HRS | SERVES: 10

INGREDIENTS:

- 3 cup dates
- ½ cup raisins
- 1½ cup raw almonds

- 4 cups raw cashews
- 1 cup unsweetened cocoa powder
- 1½ cups water

- 1 cup almond milk

DIRECTIONS:

1. Use a food processer and blend together 1 cup of dates, raisins, and almonds. They should begin to stick together. Press the date mix into a spring-form, circular pan.

2. In a blender, blend the cashews, 2 cups of dates, cocoa, water, and milk. Once thoroughly combined, pour over the crust.

3. Place the pan in the freezer for at least 2 hours, or until it doesn't jiggle when you shake it.

4. When ready to serve, take out of freezer and allow to soften just enough to cut. Store leftovers in the freezer.

CARAMEL DATE BALLS

COOK TIME: 30 MINS | SERVES: 4

INGREDIENTS:

- 1 cup dates
- 1 cup raw, unsalted cashews

- ½ cup tahini
- 1 tsp. vanilla extract

- ¼ tsp. Himalayan pink salt

DIRECTIONS:

1. First, make sure your dates are pitted.

2. Use a food processor and its chopping blade. Add the cashews and pulse until the cashews are ground finely. Put in the dates in and pulse until it all turns into a paste.

3. Mix in the tahini, vanilla, and salt. Continue pulsing. The paste should become more of a dough now. If it isn't, add a little bit of water and try again.

4. Use a tablespoon to scoop out the dough and use your hands to form the dough into balls. The mixture should be enough for about 18 balls.

5. Place the balls on a baking tray and put in the freezer. Once the balls are firm, you can put them in an airtight Tupperware and keep at room temperature.

AUTUMN APPLE BREAD

COOK TIME: 50 MINS | SERVES: 6

INGREDIENTS:

- 3 tbsp. unsweetened applesauce
- 6 tbsp. maple syrup
- 1 overripe banana
- 1 cup ground almonds
- 1 tbsp. chia seeds
- 1 cup rice flour
- Coconut oil

DIRECTIONS:

1. Preheat your oven to 390°F.

2. In a large mixing bowl, combine the applesauce, maple syrup, and peeled banana. Use a potato masher or fork to mix thoroughly.

3. Add in the ground almond, chia seeds, flour, and 4 tbsp. of water. Mix together until the batter is smooth.

4. Use coconut oil to grease a loaf-shaped tin. Use a spatula to scrape all the batter into the pan. Spread it evenly. Don't worry if the batter doesn't fill the pan up much.

5. Put in the oven and bake for about 50 minutes. It will be done when you can insert a skewer into the thickest part and pull it out clean.

6. Dump out of pan, let cool, and serve.

SUMMER FRUIT SORBET

COOK TIME: 5 MINS | SERVES: 4

INGREDIENTS:

- 2 cups frozen mango chunks
- 2 cups frozen peach chunks
- 1 cup orange juice
- Honey

DIRECTIONS:

1. Using a blender, mix together the mango, peaches, and orange juice. Blend until smooth. If it's too thick, add a little more juice or water. If you prefer a sweeter taste, add some honey.

2. You can eat it immediately, or put it in the freezer for a harder texture. Store extra in the freezer.

Quick tip: You can actually substitute the mango and peaches with any frozen fruit! You can also use any juice (or water)!

APPLE OAT COOKIES

COOK TIME: 45 MINS | SERVES: 14

INGREDIENTS:

- 10 dates
- 1 cup unsweetened applesauce
- 1 ½ teaspoons apple cider vinegar
- ¾ cup raw walnuts
- 1 cup old-fashioned oats
- ½ cup quick oatmeal
- 1 cup oat flour

- 2 tbsp. lemon zest
- 2 tsp. unsweetened cocoa powder
- 1 tsp. vanilla powder
- ½ tsp. baking soda
- Himalayan pink salt

DIRECTIONS:

Preheat your oven to 275°F and use parchment paper to line 2 baking trays.

Make sure your dates are pitted before putting them in a bowl. Fill the bowl with hot water until it covers the dates. Leave for 20 minutes.

After 20 minutes, drain the water and move the dates to a food processor. Combine with the applesauce and vinegar. Pulse until everything is combined into a smooth paste.

Roughly chop the walnuts then mix together in a large bowl both kinds of oats, the oat flour, lemon zest, cocoa powder, vanilla powder, baking soda, and a pinch of salt. Whisk together until combined.

Use a spatula to scoop out the date mixture and add to the dry ingredients. Mix well. The dough will probably be a little bit dry.

Use a muffin scoop to scoop out the dough. Use your hands to roll it into a ball, then lightly press it down on the baking tray. Do this for all of the dough.

Bake for 35-45 minutes, or until crispy and browned. Once done, cool on a wire rack before serving.

GLUTEN-FREE PEACH CRUMBLE

COOK TIME: 45 MINS | SERVES: 12

INGREDIENTS:

- 10 peaches
- ¾ cup coconut sugar
- 2 tbsp. arrowroot powder
- 3 tbsp. lemon juice
- 1 tsp. cinnamon powder
- 2 tsp. vanilla extract
- 1/8 tsp. nutmeg powder
- 1½ cups gluten-free flour
- ½ cup finely ground cornmeal
- 2 tsp. baking powder
- ½ tsp. baking soda
- ½ tsp. Himalayan pink salt
- 2/3 cup soy milk
- 1 egg
- ½ cup coconut oil
- Non-dairy vanilla ice cream

DIRECTIONS:

1. Preheat your oven to 400°F.

2. Peel and pit your peaches. Cut them into thin slices and put in a large bowl.

3. Add in ½ cup sugar, arrowroot powder, 2 tbsp. lemon juice, 1 tsp. cinnamon, 1 tsp. vanilla, and nutmeg. Mix well.

4. In a separate bowl, add the flour, cornmeal, ¼ cup sugar, baking powder, baking soda, and salt. Whisk well.

5. Mix together the milk and 2 tsp. lemon juice in a new bowl and let sit for 3 minutes.

6. Add in the egg and 1 tsp. vanilla. Whisk together until well mixed.

7. Put the coconut oil into the dry ingredients and mash together with a fork until it begins to look crumbly. Make a hole in the middle and add the liquid ingredients. Mix together just until it begins to stick.

8. Grease a 9 x 13-inch casserole dish and evenly spread the peach mixture along the bottom. Spoon the dough over top and spread evenly.

9. Put in the oven for 45 minutes. It will be done when the top is golden and crispy and the peaches are bubbling.

10. Let cool slightly before serving with vanilla ice cream.

RAISIN ALMOND OATMEAL COOKIES

COOK TIME: 15 MINS | SERVES: 24

INGREDIENTS:

- 1 cup whole wheat flour
- 1 tsp. cinnamon powder
- ½ tsp. baking powder
- ½ tsp. baking soda
- ½ tsp. Himalayan pink salt
- ¼ tsp. nutmeg powder
- ½ cup coconut oil

- ⅓ cup almond butter
- ½ cup honey
- 1 overripe banana
- 1 tsp. vanilla extract
- 1½ cups old-fashioned oats
- ¾ cup raisins

DIRECTIONS:

Preheat your oven to 350°F. Prep two baking trays by placing parchment paper on top.

Combine in a large bowl the flour, cinnamon, baking powder, baking soda, salt, and nutmeg. Whisk together until combined.

In the bowl of a stand mixer, add the oil, almond butter, honey, banana, and vanilla. Use the paddle attachment and beat until combined.

Pour in the dry ingredients slowly and beat lightly until mixed in. Add the oats and raisins. Beat again until mixed.

Put the dough in the refrigerator until it is firm.

Use a tablespoon to scoop the dough into rounds onto the baking trays, leaving space between each one. Press the dough balls down to make them a little flatter.

Bake for 10-12 minutes, depending on your preference of crispness.

Before serving, allow the cookies to cool on a cooling rack.

BLUEBERRY COCONUT MILKSHAKE

COOK TIME: 5 MINS | SERVES: 2

INGREDIENTS:

- 1 can coconut milk
- 1½ cups frozen blueberries
- 1 tbsp. honey
- 1 tsp. vanilla extract

DIRECTIONS:

1. Use a blender to mix together all the ingredients until smooth. If it's too thick, add a little water. Serve immediately.

Quick tip: You can use any kind of milk if you don't like coconut milk. You could also use other frozen fruit. If you want it extra thick, try adding cashew butter!

CASHEW LEMON DROPS

COOK TIME: 1 HR | SERVES: 20

INGREDIENTS:

- ½ cup raw cashews
- 2 tbsp. honey
- 2 tbsp. lemon juice
- ½ cup coconut oil
- Himalayan pink salt

DIRECTIONS:

1. Line a baking tray with wax paper and put it in the freezer.
2. Use a food processor to pulse the cashews several times until they are ground finely.
3. Mix in the honey and lemon juice before pulsing again.
4. Mix in the oil and a pinch of salt, then continue to pulse until pureed.
5. Take the baking tray from the freezer and spoon small chunks of the puree onto the tray.
6. Put the tray back in the freezer for an hour, or until the chunks are hard.
7. Serve cold and store the leftovers in the freezer.

HAZELNUT CHOC PUDDING

COOK TIME: 5 MINS | SERVES: 2

INGREDIENTS:

- 1 avocado
- 2 tbsp. raw cacao powder
- 1 tbsp. honey
- 1 tsp. vanilla extract
- Himalayan pink salt
- 2 tbsp. hazelnuts

DIRECTIONS:

1. Half and pit the avocado, then put it into a food processor. Add the cacao, honey, vanilla, and a pinch of salt. Pulse until it becomes a thick puree.

2. Split the mixture into two bowls and leave in the fridge if not serving immediately. Before serving, chop the hazelnuts and sprinkle on top.

COCONUT CHIA BLUEBERRY PUDDING

COOK TIME: 8 HRS | SERVES: 4

INGREDIENTS:

- ½ cup chia seeds
- 2 cups almond milk
- 2 tbsp. honey
- 1½ tsp. vanilla extract
- ¼ tsp. sea salt
- 2 cups blueberries
- ¼ cup shredded coconut

DIRECTIONS:

1. Mix together in a bowl the chia seeds, milk, honey, vanilla, and salt. Leave the bowl to stand for 15 minutes. Mix again to avoid large chunks and cover with a lid. Put in the fridge for a minimum of 8 hours.

2. Before serving, feel free to add more milk if it's too thick.

3. To serve, garnish each bowl of pudding with ½ cup of blueberries and a sprinkle of coconut. If desired, swirl a little honey on top as well.

Quick tip: You can replace the blueberries with any fruit and it will be just as delicious!

CPSIA information can be obtained
at www.ICGtesting.com
Printed in the USA
BVHW010847020821
613408BV00003B/108